List all medications and time of day

Name of Medication	Dosage	Fre	

List all medications and time of day you take them

Name of Medication	Dosage	Frequency	Time of Day

List all medications and time of day you take them

Name of Medication	Dosage	Frequency	Time of Day

For your wallet/purse:

| **I Have Parkinson's Disease** | Contacts: |

For your wallet/purse:

| **Meds** | **Meds** |

BLANK PAGE

Date: 1/4/22   **Daily Log**   Overall Rating: 😊 (😐) ☹

Did you remember to take your medications today?	Off times: Time of day symptoms started: _____
7/9:30 am/pm y/n 12 am/pm y/n 4 am/pm y/n 7 am/pm y/n 11 am/pm y/n	Symptoms: (Fatigue), (Tremors), Mood Change, Sweating, Anxiety, Not Thinking Clearly, Feeling Restless (circle any that apply) Other _____

Evaluate your sleep last night.
Scale : 0 1 2 ③ 4 5 (poor 0 to excellent 5)
Bad or disturbing dreams? _____no_____

Dizziness? y/n _____no_____
Falls? y/n _____no_____
Depression? y/n _____no_____   Alcohol? y/n
Hallucinations? y/n _____no_____   How much? ___no___

Did you exercise today? y/n How Long? __5__ minutes
Type of Exercise: _____WALKING_____

Did you eat three balanced healthy meals today?
Breakfast y/n _____yes_____
Lunch y/n _____yes_____
Dinner y/n _____yes_____

What did you accomplish today? _____
_____

Date: 2/4/22 **Daily Log** Overall Rating: 😀 😐 ☹

Did you remember to take your medications today?

_____am/pm y/n
_____am/pm y/n
_____am/pm y/n
_____am/pm y/n
_____am/pm y/n

Off times: Time of day symptoms started: _____

Symptoms: Fatigue, Tremors, Mood Change, Sweating, Anxiety, Not Thinking Clearly, Feeling Restless (circle any that apply)
Other _____

Evaluate your sleep last night.
Scale : 0 1 2 3 4 5 (poor 0 to excellent 5)
Bad or disturbing dreams?_____

Dizziness? y/n _____
Falls? y/n _____
Depression? y/n _____   Alcohol? y/n
Hallucinations? y/n _____   How much?_____

Did you exercise today? y/n How Long? _____ minutes
Type of Exercise: _____

Did you eat three balanced healthy meals today?
Breakfast y/n _____
Lunch y/n _____
Dinner y/n _____

What did you accomplish today? _____
_____

Date: 3/4/22   **Daily Log**   Overall Rating: ☺ 😐 ☹

| Did you remember to take your medications today?

_____am/pm y/n
_____am/pm y/n
_____am/pm y/n
_____am/pm y/n
_____am/pm y/n | Off times: Time of day symptoms started: _____

Symptoms: Fatigue, Tremors, Mood Change, Sweating, Anxiety, Not Thinking Clearly, Feeling Restless (circle any that apply)
Other _____ |

Evaluate your sleep last night.
Scale : 0 1 2 3 4 5 (poor 0 to excellent 5)
Bad or disturbing dreams?_____

Dizziness? y/n _____
Falls? y/n _____
Depression? y/n _____   Alcohol? y/n
Hallucinations? y/n _____   How much?_____

Did you exercise today? y/n How Long? _____ minutes
Type of Exercise: _____

Did you eat three balanced healthy meals today?
Breakfast y/n _____
Lunch y/n _____
Dinner y/n _____

What did you accomplish today? _____
_____

Date: 4/4/22   **Daily Log**   Overall Rating: 😊 😐 ☹️

Did you remember to take your medications today?

_____am/pm y/n
_____am/pm y/n
_____am/pm y/n
_____am/pm y/n
_____am/pm y/n

Off times: Time of day symptoms started: _____

Symptoms: Fatigue, Tremors, Mood Change, Sweating, Anxiety, Not Thinking Clearly, Feeling Restless (circle any that apply)
Other _____

Evaluate your sleep last night.
Scale : 0 1 2 3 4 5 (poor 0 to excellent 5)
Bad or disturbing dreams?_____

Dizziness? y/n _____
Falls? y/n _____
Depression? y/n _____   Alcohol? y/n
Hallucinations? y/n _____   How much?_____

Did you exercise today? y/n How Long? _____ minutes
Type of Exercise: _____

Did you eat three balanced healthy meals today?
Breakfast y/n _____
Lunch y/n _____
Dinner y/n _____

What did you accomplish today? _____
_____

Date: 5/4/22   **Daily Log**   Overall Rating: 😊 😐 ☹

Did you remember to take your medications today?	Off times: Time of day symptoms started: _____
7/9:30 am/pm **y**/n 12 am/pm **y**/n 4 am/pm **y**/n 7 am/pm **y**/n 11 am/pm **y**/n	Symptoms: Fatigue, **Tremors**, Mood Change, Sweating, Anxiety, Not Thinking Clearly, Feeling Restless (circle any that apply) Other _____

Evaluate your sleep last night.
Scale : 0 1 2 3 4 5 (poor 0 to excellent 5)
Bad or disturbing dreams? _____

Dizziness? y/n _____
Falls? y/n _____
Depression? y/n _____   Alcohol? y/n
Hallucinations? y/n _____   How much? _____

Did you exercise today? y/n How Long? _____ minutes
Type of Exercise: _____

Did you eat three balanced healthy meals today?
Breakfast y/n _____
Lunch y/n _____
Dinner y/n _____

What did you accomplish today? _____
_____

Date: 6/4/22   **Daily Log**   Overall Rating: ☺ 😐 ☹

Did you remember to take your medications today?

7 / 9:30	am/pm	y/n
12	am/pm	y/n
4	am/pm	y/n
7	am/pm	y/n
11	am/pm	y/n

Off times: Time of day symptoms started: _____

Symptoms: (Fatigue), (Tremors), Mood Change, Sweating, Anxiety, Not Thinking Clearly, Feeling Restless (circle any that apply)
Other _____

Evaluate your sleep last night.
Scale: 0 1 2 ③ 4 5 (poor 0 to excellent 5)
Bad or disturbing dreams? _____

Dizziness? y/n ___no___
Falls? y/n ___no___
Depression? y/n ___no___   Alcohol? y/n
Hallucinations? y/n ___no___   How much? ___no___

Did you exercise today? y/n   How Long? __5__ minutes
Type of Exercise: ___walking___

Did you eat three balanced healthy meals today?
Breakfast y/n ___yes___
Lunch y/n ___yes___
Dinner y/n ___yes___

What did you accomplish today? ___Some cleaning___
___Large Text panel running 2 lines___

Date: 7/4/22 **Daily Log** Overall Rating: 😊 😐 ☹️

Did you remember to take your medications today?

7 9:30 am/pm	(y)/n
12 am/pm	(y)/n
4 am/pm	y/n
7 am/pm	y/n
11 am/pm	y/n

Off times: Time of day symptoms started: _____

Symptoms: Fatigue, Tremors, Mood Change, Sweating, Anxiety, Not Thinking Clearly, Feeling Restless (circle any that apply)
Other _____

Evaluate your sleep last night.
Scale: 0 1 2 ③ 4 5 (poor 0 to excellent 5)
Bad or disturbing dreams? _____ no _____

Dizziness? y/n _____
Falls? y/n _____
Depression? y/n _____ Alcohol? y/n
Hallucinations? y/n _____ How much? _____

Did you exercise today? y/n How Long? _____ minutes
Type of Exercise: _____

Did you eat three balanced healthy meals today?
Breakfast (y)/n _____ w/oatabrya _____
Lunch y/n _____
Dinner y/n _____

What did you accomplish today? _____
_____

Date:_____   **Daily Log**   Overall Rating: ☺ 😐 ☹

| Did you remember to take your medications today?

_____am/pm y/n
_____am/pm y/n
_____am/pm y/n
_____am/pm y/n
_____am/pm y/n | Off times: Time of day symptoms started: _____

Symptoms: Fatigue, Tremors, Mood Change, Sweating, Anxiety, Not Thinking Clearly, Feeling Restless (circle any that apply)
Other _____ |

Evaluate your sleep last night.
Scale : 0 1 2 3 4 5 (poor 0 to excellent 5)
Bad or disturbing dreams?_____

Dizziness? y/n _____
Falls? y/n _____
Depression? y/n _____   Alcohol? y/n
Hallucinations? y/n _____   How much?_____

Did you exercise today? y/n How Long? _____ minutes
Type of Exercise: _____

Did you eat three balanced healthy meals today?
Breakfast y/n _____
Lunch y/n _____
Dinner y/n _____

What did you accomplish today? _____
_____

Date:_____ **Daily Log**   Overall Rating: 😊 😐 ☹

| Did you remember to take your medications today?

_____am/pm y/n
_____am/pm y/n
_____am/pm y/n
_____am/pm y/n
_____am/pm y/n | Off times: Time of day symptoms started: _____

Symptoms: Fatigue, Tremors, Mood Change, Sweating, Anxiety, Not Thinking Clearly, Feeling Restless (circle any that apply)
Other _____ |

Evaluate your sleep last night.
Scale : 0 1 2 3 4 5 (poor 0 to excellent 5)
Bad or disturbing dreams?_____

Dizziness? y/n _____
Falls? y/n _____
Depression? y/n _____   Alcohol? y/n
Hallucinations? y/n _____   How much?_____

Did you exercise today? y/n How Long? _____ minutes
Type of Exercise: _____

Did you eat three balanced healthy meals today?
Breakfast y/n _____
Lunch y/n _____
Dinner y/n _____

What did you accomplish today? _____
_____

Date:_____ **Daily Log** Overall Rating: 😊 😐 ☹️

| Did you remember to take your medications today?

_____am/pm y/n
_____am/pm y/n
_____am/pm y/n
_____am/pm y/n
_____am/pm y/n | Off times: Time of day symptoms started: _____

Symptoms: Fatigue, Tremors, Mood Change, Sweating, Anxiety, Not Thinking Clearly, Feeling Restless (circle any that apply)
Other _____ |

Evaluate your sleep last night.
Scale : 0 1 2 3 4 5 (poor 0 to excellent 5)
Bad or disturbing dreams?_____

Dizziness? y/n _____
Falls? y/n _____
Depression? y/n _____   Alcohol? y/n
Hallucinations? y/n _____   How much?_____

Did you exercise today? y/n How Long? _____ minutes
Type of Exercise: _____

Did you eat three balanced healthy meals today?
Breakfast y/n _____
Lunch y/n _____
Dinner y/n _____

What did you accomplish today? _____
_____

Date:_____ **Daily Log** Overall Rating: 😊 😐 ☹

Did you remember to take your medications today?	Off times: Time of day symptoms started: _____
_____am/pm y/n _____am/pm y/n _____am/pm y/n _____am/pm y/n _____am/pm y/n	Symptoms: Fatigue, Tremors, Mood Change, Sweating, Anxiety, Not Thinking Clearly, Feeling Restless (circle any that apply) Other _____

Evaluate your sleep last night.
Scale : 0 1 2 3 4 5 (poor 0 to excellent 5)
Bad or disturbing dreams?_____

Dizziness? y/n _____
Falls? y/n _____
Depression? y/n _____   Alcohol? y/n
Hallucinations? y/n _____   How much?_____

Did you exercise today? y/n How Long? _____ minutes
Type of Exercise: _____

Did you eat three balanced healthy meals today?
Breakfast y/n _____
Lunch y/n _____
Dinner y/n _____

What did you accomplish today? _____
_____

Date:_____ **Daily Log** Overall Rating: 😊 😐 ☹️

| Did you remember to take your medications today?

_____am/pm y/n
_____am/pm y/n
_____am/pm y/n
_____am/pm y/n
_____am/pm y/n | Off times: Time of day symptoms started: _____

Symptoms: Fatigue, Tremors, Mood Change, Sweating, Anxiety, Not Thinking Clearly, Feeling Restless (circle any that apply)
Other _____ |

Evaluate your sleep last night.
Scale : 0 1 2 3 4 5 (poor 0 to excellent 5)
Bad or disturbing dreams?_____

Dizziness? y/n _____
Falls? y/n _____
Depression? y/n _____   Alcohol? y/n
Hallucinations? y/n _____   How much?_____

Did you exercise today? y/n How Long? _____ minutes
Type of Exercise: _____

Did you eat three balanced healthy meals today?
Breakfast y/n _____
Lunch y/n _____
Dinner y/n _____

What did you accomplish today? _____
_____

Date:_____ **Daily Log** Overall Rating: 😀 😐 ☹

Did you remember to take your medications today?

_____am/pm y/n
_____am/pm y/n
_____am/pm y/n
_____am/pm y/n
_____am/pm y/n

Off times: Time of day symptoms started: _____

Symptoms: Fatigue, Tremors, Mood Change, Sweating, Anxiety, Not Thinking Clearly, Feeling Restless (circle any that apply)
Other _____

Evaluate your sleep last night.
Scale : 0 1 2 3 4 5 (poor 0 to excellent 5)
Bad or disturbing dreams?_____

Dizziness? y/n _____
Falls? y/n _____
Depression? y/n _____ Alcohol? y/n
Hallucinations? y/n _____ How much?_____

Did you exercise today? y/n How Long? _____ minutes
Type of Exercise: _____

Did you eat three balanced healthy meals today?
Breakfast y/n _____
Lunch y/n _____
Dinner y/n _____

What did you accomplish today? _____
_____

Date:_____ **Daily Log** Overall Rating: 😊 😐 ☹

| Did you remember to take your medications today?

_____am/pm y/n
_____am/pm y/n
_____am/pm y/n
_____am/pm y/n
_____am/pm y/n | Off times: Time of day symptoms started: _____

Symptoms: Fatigue, Tremors, Mood Change, Sweating, Anxiety, Not Thinking Clearly, Feeling Restless (circle any that apply)
Other _____ |

Evaluate your sleep last night.
Scale : 0 1 2 3 4 5   (poor 0 to excellent 5)
Bad or disturbing dreams?_____

Dizziness? y/n _____
Falls? y/n _____
Depression? y/n _____   Alcohol? y/n
Hallucinations? y/n _____   How much?_____

Did you exercise today? y/n How Long? _____ minutes
Type of Exercise: _____

Did you eat three balanced healthy meals today?
Breakfast y/n _____
Lunch y/n _____
Dinner y/n _____

What did you accomplish today? _____
_____

Date:_____ **Daily Log** Overall Rating: 😊 😐 ☹️

Did you remember to take your medications today?

_____am/pm y/n
_____am/pm y/n
_____am/pm y/n
_____am/pm y/n
_____am/pm y/n

Off times: Time of day symptoms started: _____

Symptoms: Fatigue, Tremors, Mood Change, Sweating, Anxiety, Not Thinking Clearly, Feeling Restless (circle any that apply)
Other _____

Evaluate your sleep last night.
Scale : 0 1 2 3 4 5 (poor 0 to excellent 5)
Bad or disturbing dreams?_____

Dizziness? y/n _____
Falls? y/n _____
Depression? y/n _____   Alcohol? y/n
Hallucinations? y/n _____   How much?_____

Did you exercise today? y/n How Long? _____ minutes
Type of Exercise: _____

Did you eat three balanced healthy meals today?
Breakfast y/n _____
Lunch y/n _____
Dinner y/n _____

What did you accomplish today? _____
_____

Date:_____ **Daily Log** Overall Rating: 😊 😐 ☹️

| Did you remember to take your medications today?

_____am/pm y/n
_____am/pm y/n
_____am/pm y/n
_____am/pm y/n
_____am/pm y/n | Off times: Time of day symptoms started: _____

Symptoms: Fatigue, Tremors, Mood Change, Sweating, Anxiety, Not Thinking Clearly, Feeling Restless (circle any that apply)
Other _____ |

Evaluate your sleep last night.
Scale : 0 1 2 3 4 5 (poor 0 to excellent 5)
Bad or disturbing dreams?_____

Dizziness? y/n _____
Falls? y/n _____
Depression? y/n _____   Alcohol? y/n
Hallucinations? y/n _____   How much?_____

Did you exercise today? y/n How Long? _____ minutes
Type of Exercise: _____

Did you eat three balanced healthy meals today?
Breakfast y/n _____
Lunch y/n _____
Dinner y/n _____

What did you accomplish today? _____
_____

Date:_____ **Daily Log** Overall Rating: 😊 😐 ☹

Did you remember to take your medications today?	Off times: Time of day symptoms started: _____
_____am/pm y/n _____am/pm y/n _____am/pm y/n _____am/pm y/n _____am/pm y/n	Symptoms: Fatigue, Tremors, Mood Change, Sweating, Anxiety, Not Thinking Clearly, Feeling Restless (circle any that apply) Other _____

Evaluate your sleep last night.
Scale : 0 1 2 3 4 5 (poor 0 to excellent 5)
Bad or disturbing dreams?_____

Dizziness? y/n _____
Falls? y/n _____
Depression? y/n _____   Alcohol? y/n
Hallucinations? y/n _____   How much?_____

Did you exercise today? y/n How Long? _____ minutes
Type of Exercise: _____

Did you eat three balanced healthy meals today?
Breakfast y/n _____
Lunch y/n _____
Dinner y/n _____

What did you accomplish today? _____
_____

Date:_____   **Daily Log**   Overall Rating: ☺ 😐 ☹

| Did you remember to take your medications today?

_____am/pm y/n
_____am/pm y/n
_____am/pm y/n
_____am/pm y/n
_____am/pm y/n | Off times: Time of day symptoms started: _____

Symptoms: Fatigue, Tremors, Mood Change, Sweating, Anxiety, Not Thinking Clearly, Feeling Restless (circle any that apply)
Other _____ |

Evaluate your sleep last night.
Scale : 0 1 2 3 4 5 (poor 0 to excellent 5)
Bad or disturbing dreams?_____

Dizziness? y/n _____
Falls? y/n _____
Depression? y/n _____   Alcohol? y/n
Hallucinations? y/n _____   How much?_____

Did you exercise today? y/n How Long? _____ minutes
Type of Exercise: _____

Did you eat three balanced healthy meals today?
Breakfast y/n _____
Lunch y/n _____
Dinner y/n _____

What did you accomplish today? _____
_____

Date:_____   **Daily Log**   Overall Rating: ☺ 😐 ☹

| Did you remember to take your medications today?

_____am/pm y/n
_____am/pm y/n
_____am/pm y/n
_____am/pm y/n
_____am/pm y/n | Off times: Time of day symptoms started: _____

Symptoms: Fatigue, Tremors, Mood Change, Sweating, Anxiety, Not Thinking Clearly, Feeling Restless (circle any that apply)
Other _____ |

Evaluate your sleep last night.
Scale : 0 1 2 3 4 5 (poor 0 to excellent 5)
Bad or disturbing dreams?_____

Dizziness? y/n _____
Falls? y/n _____
Depression? y/n _____   Alcohol? y/n
Hallucinations? y/n _____   How much?_____

Did you exercise today? y/n How Long? _____ minutes
Type of Exercise: _____

Did you eat three balanced healthy meals today?
Breakfast y/n _____
Lunch y/n _____
Dinner y/n _____

What did you accomplish today? _____
_____

Date:_____   **Daily Log**   Overall Rating: 😊 😐 ☹

| Did you remember to take your medications today? _____am/pm y/n _____am/pm y/n _____am/pm y/n _____am/pm y/n _____am/pm y/n | Off times: Time of day symptoms started: _____ Symptoms: Fatigue, Tremors, Mood Change, Sweating, Anxiety, Not Thinking Clearly, Feeling Restless (circle any that apply) Other _____ |

Evaluate your sleep last night.
Scale : 0 1 2 3 4 5   (poor 0 to excellent 5)
Bad or disturbing dreams?_____

Dizziness? y/n _____
Falls? y/n _____
Depression? y/n _____   Alcohol? y/n
Hallucinations? y/n _____   How much?_____

Did you exercise today? y/n How Long? _____ minutes
Type of Exercise: _____

Did you eat three balanced healthy meals today?
Breakfast y/n _____
Lunch y/n _____
Dinner y/n _____

What did you accomplish today? _____
_____

Date:_____ **Daily Log** Overall Rating: 😊 😐 ☹

| Did you remember to take your medications today?

_____am/pm y/n
_____am/pm y/n
_____am/pm y/n
_____am/pm y/n
_____am/pm y/n | Off times: Time of day symptoms started: _____

Symptoms: Fatigue, Tremors, Mood Change, Sweating, Anxiety, Not Thinking Clearly, Feeling Restless (circle any that apply)
Other _____ |

Evaluate your sleep last night.
Scale : 0 1 2 3 4 5   (poor 0 to excellent 5)
Bad or disturbing dreams?_____

Dizziness? y/n _____
Falls? y/n _____
Depression? y/n _____   Alcohol? y/n
Hallucinations? y/n _____   How much?_____

Did you exercise today? y/n How Long? _____ minutes
Type of Exercise: _____

Did you eat three balanced healthy meals today?
Breakfast y/n _____
Lunch y/n _____
Dinner y/n _____

What did you accomplish today? _____
_____

Date:_____ **Daily Log**   Overall Rating: ☺ 😐 ☹

| Did you remember to take your medications today?

_____am/pm y/n
_____am/pm y/n
_____am/pm y/n
_____am/pm y/n
_____am/pm y/n | Off times: Time of day symptoms started: _____

Symptoms: Fatigue, Tremors, Mood Change, Sweating, Anxiety, Not Thinking Clearly, Feeling Restless (circle any that apply)
Other _____ |

Evaluate your sleep last night.
Scale : 0 1 2 3 4 5 (poor 0 to excellent 5)
Bad or disturbing dreams?_____

Dizziness? y/n _____
Falls? y/n _____
Depression? y/n _____   Alcohol? y/n
Hallucinations? y/n _____   How much?_____

Did you exercise today? y/n How Long? _____ minutes
Type of Exercise: _____

Did you eat three balanced healthy meals today?
Breakfast y/n _____
Lunch y/n _____
Dinner y/n _____

What did you accomplish today? _____
_____

Date:_____   **Daily Log**   Overall Rating: 😊 😐 ☹

| Did you remember to take your medications today?

_____am/pm y/n
_____am/pm y/n
_____am/pm y/n
_____am/pm y/n
_____am/pm y/n | Off times: Time of day symptoms started: _____

Symptoms: Fatigue, Tremors, Mood Change, Sweating, Anxiety, Not Thinking Clearly, Feeling Restless (circle any that apply)
Other _____ |

Evaluate your sleep last night.
Scale : 0 1 2 3 4 5 (poor 0 to excellent 5)
Bad or disturbing dreams?_____

Dizziness? y/n _____
Falls? y/n _____
Depression? y/n _____   Alcohol? y/n
Hallucinations? y/n _____   How much?_____

Did you exercise today? y/n How Long? _____ minutes
Type of Exercise: _____

Did you eat three balanced healthy meals today?
Breakfast y/n _____
Lunch y/n _____
Dinner y/n _____

What did you accomplish today? _____
_____

Date:_____ **Daily Log**   Overall Rating: ☺ 😐 ☹

| Did you remember to take your medications today?

_____am/pm y/n
_____am/pm y/n
_____am/pm y/n
_____am/pm y/n
_____am/pm y/n | Off times: Time of day symptoms started: _____

Symptoms: Fatigue, Tremors, Mood Change, Sweating, Anxiety, Not Thinking Clearly, Feeling Restless (circle any that apply)
Other _____ |

Evaluate your sleep last night.
Scale : 0 1 2 3 4 5   (poor 0 to excellent 5)
Bad or disturbing dreams?_____

Dizziness? y/n _____
Falls? y/n _____
Depression? y/n _____   Alcohol? y/n
Hallucinations? y/n _____   How much?_____

Did you exercise today? y/n How Long? _____ minutes
Type of Exercise: _____

Did you eat three balanced healthy meals today?
Breakfast y/n _____
Lunch y/n _____
Dinner y/n _____

What did you accomplish today? _____
_____

Date:_____   **Daily Log**   Overall Rating: 😊 😐 ☹

| Did you remember to take your medications today?

_____am/pm y/n
_____am/pm y/n
_____am/pm y/n
_____am/pm y/n
_____am/pm y/n | Off times: Time of day symptoms started: _____

Symptoms: Fatigue, Tremors, Mood Change, Sweating, Anxiety, Not Thinking Clearly, Feeling Restless (circle any that apply)
Other _____ |

Evaluate your sleep last night.
Scale : 0 1 2 3 4 5 (poor 0 to excellent 5)
Bad or disturbing dreams?_____

Dizziness? y/n _____
Falls? y/n _____
Depression? y/n _____   Alcohol? y/n
Hallucinations? y/n _____   How much?_____

Did you exercise today? y/n How Long? _____ minutes
Type of Exercise: _____

Did you eat three balanced healthy meals today?
Breakfast y/n _____
Lunch y/n _____
Dinner y/n _____

What did you accomplish today? _____
_____

Date:_____ **Daily Log** Overall Rating: ☺ 😐 ☹

Did you remember to take your medications today? _____am/pm y/n _____am/pm y/n _____am/pm y/n _____am/pm y/n _____am/pm y/n	Off times: Time of day symptoms started: _____ Symptoms: Fatigue, Tremors, Mood Change, Sweating, Anxiety, Not Thinking Clearly, Feeling Restless (circle any that apply) Other _____

Evaluate your sleep last night.
Scale : 0 1 2 3 4 5   (poor 0 to excellent 5)
Bad or disturbing dreams?_____

Dizziness? y/n _____
Falls? y/n _____
Depression? y/n _____   Alcohol? y/n
Hallucinations? y/n _____   How much?_____

Did you exercise today? y/n How Long? _____ minutes
Type of Exercise: _____

Did you eat three balanced healthy meals today?
Breakfast y/n _____
Lunch y/n _____
Dinner y/n _____

What did you accomplish today? _____
_____

Date:_____ **Daily Log** Overall Rating: 😊 😐 ☹

| Did you remember to take your medications today?

_____am/pm y/n
_____am/pm y/n
_____am/pm y/n
_____am/pm y/n
_____am/pm y/n | Off times: Time of day symptoms started: _____

Symptoms: Fatigue, Tremors, Mood Change, Sweating, Anxiety, Not Thinking Clearly, Feeling Restless (circle any that apply)
Other _____ |

Evaluate your sleep last night.
Scale : 0 1 2 3 4 5 (poor 0 to excellent 5)
Bad or disturbing dreams?_____

Dizziness? y/n _____
Falls? y/n _____
Depression? y/n _____ Alcohol? y/n
Hallucinations? y/n _____ How much?_____

Did you exercise today? y/n How Long? _____ minutes
Type of Exercise: _____

Did you eat three balanced healthy meals today?
Breakfast y/n _____
Lunch y/n _____
Dinner y/n _____

What did you accomplish today? _____
_____

Date:_____ **Daily Log** Overall Rating: 😊 😐 ☹️

Did you remember to take your medications today?	Off times: Time of day symptoms started: _____
_____am/pm y/n _____am/pm y/n _____am/pm y/n _____am/pm y/n _____am/pm y/n	Symptoms: Fatigue, Tremors, Mood Change, Sweating, Anxiety, Not Thinking Clearly, Feeling Restless (circle any that apply) Other _____

Evaluate your sleep last night.
Scale : 0 1 2 3 4 5   (poor 0 to excellent 5)
Bad or disturbing dreams?_____

Dizziness? y/n _____
Falls? y/n _____
Depression? y/n _____   Alcohol? y/n
Hallucinations? y/n _____   How much?_____

Did you exercise today? y/n How Long? _____ minutes
Type of Exercise: _____

Did you eat three balanced healthy meals today?
Breakfast y/n _____
Lunch y/n _____
Dinner y/n _____

What did you accomplish today? _____
_____

Date:_____ **Daily Log** Overall Rating: 😊 😐 ☹

| Did you remember to take your medications today?

_____am/pm y/n
_____am/pm y/n
_____am/pm y/n
_____am/pm y/n
_____am/pm y/n | Off times: Time of day symptoms started: _____

Symptoms: Fatigue, Tremors, Mood Change, Sweating, Anxiety, Not Thinking Clearly, Feeling Restless (circle any that apply)
Other _____ |

Evaluate your sleep last night.
Scale : 0 1 2 3 4 5 (poor 0 to excellent 5)
Bad or disturbing dreams?_____

Dizziness? y/n _____
Falls? y/n _____
Depression? y/n _____ Alcohol? y/n
Hallucinations? y/n _____ How much?_____

Did you exercise today? y/n How Long? _____ minutes
Type of Exercise: _____

Did you eat three balanced healthy meals today?
Breakfast y/n _____
Lunch y/n _____
Dinner y/n _____

What did you accomplish today? _____
_____

Date:_____ **Daily Log** Overall Rating: 😊 😐 ☹️

| Did you remember to take your medications today?

_____am/pm y/n
_____am/pm y/n
_____am/pm y/n
_____am/pm y/n
_____am/pm y/n | Off times: Time of day symptoms started: _____

Symptoms: Fatigue, Tremors, Mood Change, Sweating, Anxiety, Not Thinking Clearly, Feeling Restless (circle any that apply)
Other _____ |

Evaluate your sleep last night.
Scale : 0 1 2 3 4 5 (poor 0 to excellent 5)
Bad or disturbing dreams?_____

Dizziness? y/n _____
Falls? y/n _____
Depression? y/n _____   Alcohol? y/n
Hallucinations? y/n _____   How much?_____

Did you exercise today? y/n How Long? _____ minutes
Type of Exercise: _____

Did you eat three balanced healthy meals today?
Breakfast y/n _____
Lunch y/n _____
Dinner y/n _____

What did you accomplish today? _____
_____

Date:_____ **Daily Log** Overall Rating: 🙂 😐 ☹️

| Did you remember to take your medications today?

_____am/pm y/n
_____am/pm y/n
_____am/pm y/n
_____am/pm y/n
_____am/pm y/n | Off times: Time of day symptoms started: _____

Symptoms: Fatigue, Tremors, Mood Change, Sweating, Anxiety, Not Thinking Clearly, Feeling Restless (circle any that apply)
Other _____ |

Evaluate your sleep last night.
Scale : 0 1 2 3 4 5 (poor 0 to excellent 5)
Bad or disturbing dreams?_____

Dizziness? y/n _____
Falls? y/n _____
Depression? y/n _____   Alcohol? y/n
Hallucinations? y/n _____   How much?_____

Did you exercise today? y/n How Long? _____ minutes
Type of Exercise: _____

Did you eat three balanced healthy meals today?
Breakfast y/n _____
Lunch y/n _____
Dinner y/n _____

What did you accomplish today? _____
_____

Date:_____ **Daily Log**   Overall Rating: 😊 😐 ☹

| Did you remember to take your medications today?

_____am/pm y/n
_____am/pm y/n
_____am/pm y/n
_____am/pm y/n
_____am/pm y/n | Off times: Time of day symptoms started: _____

Symptoms: Fatigue, Tremors, Mood Change, Sweating, Anxiety, Not Thinking Clearly, Feeling Restless (circle any that apply)
Other _____ |

Evaluate your sleep last night.
Scale : 0 1 2 3 4 5   (poor 0 to excellent 5)
Bad or disturbing dreams?_____

Dizziness? y/n _____
Falls? y/n _____
Depression? y/n _____   Alcohol? y/n
Hallucinations? y/n _____   How much?_____

Did you exercise today? y/n How Long? _____ minutes
Type of Exercise: _____

Did you eat three balanced healthy meals today?
Breakfast y/n _____
Lunch y/n _____
Dinner y/n _____

What did you accomplish today? _____
_____

Date:_____ **Daily Log** Overall Rating: 😊 😐 ☹

Did you remember to take your medications today?

_____am/pm y/n
_____am/pm y/n
_____am/pm y/n
_____am/pm y/n
_____am/pm y/n

Off times: Time of day symptoms started: _____

Symptoms: Fatigue, Tremors, Mood Change, Sweating, Anxiety, Not Thinking Clearly, Feeling Restless (circle any that apply)
Other _____

Evaluate your sleep last night.
Scale : 0 1 2 3 4 5 (poor 0 to excellent 5)
Bad or disturbing dreams?_____

Dizziness? y/n _____
Falls? y/n _____
Depression? y/n _____   Alcohol? y/n
Hallucinations? y/n _____   How much?_____

Did you exercise today? y/n How Long? _____ minutes
Type of Exercise: _____

Did you eat three balanced healthy meals today?
Breakfast y/n _____
Lunch y/n _____
Dinner y/n _____

What did you accomplish today? _____
_____

Date:_____ **Daily Log**   Overall Rating: ☺ 😐 ☹

Did you remember to take your medications today?

_____am/pm y/n
_____am/pm y/n
_____am/pm y/n
_____am/pm y/n
_____am/pm y/n

Off times: Time of day symptoms started: _____

Symptoms: Fatigue, Tremors, Mood Change, Sweating, Anxiety, Not Thinking Clearly, Feeling Restless (circle any that apply)
Other _____

Evaluate your sleep last night.
Scale : 0 1 2 3 4 5 (poor 0 to excellent 5)
Bad or disturbing dreams?_____

Dizziness? y/n _____
Falls? y/n _____
Depression? y/n _____   Alcohol? y/n
Hallucinations? y/n _____   How much?_____

Did you exercise today? y/n How Long? _____ minutes
Type of Exercise: _____

Did you eat three balanced healthy meals today?
Breakfast y/n _____
Lunch y/n _____
Dinner y/n _____

What did you accomplish today? _____
_____

Date:_____ **Daily Log** Overall Rating: 😊 😐 ☹️

| Did you remember to take your medications today?

_____ am/pm y/n
_____ am/pm y/n
_____ am/pm y/n
_____ am/pm y/n
_____ am/pm y/n | Off times: Time of day symptoms started: _____

Symptoms: Fatigue, Tremors, Mood Change, Sweating, Anxiety, Not Thinking Clearly, Feeling Restless (circle any that apply)
Other _____ |

Evaluate your sleep last night.
Scale : 0 1 2 3 4 5 (poor 0 to excellent 5)
Bad or disturbing dreams?_____

Dizziness? y/n _____
Falls? y/n _____
Depression? y/n _____   Alcohol? y/n
Hallucinations? y/n _____   How much?_____

Did you exercise today? y/n How Long? _____ minutes
Type of Exercise: _____

Did you eat three balanced healthy meals today?
Breakfast y/n _____
Lunch y/n _____
Dinner y/n _____

What did you accomplish today? _____
_____

Date:_____ **Daily Log** Overall Rating: 😊 😐 ☹

| Did you remember to take your medications today?

_____am/pm y/n
_____am/pm y/n
_____am/pm y/n
_____am/pm y/n
_____am/pm y/n | Off times: Time of day symptoms started: _____

Symptoms: Fatigue, Tremors, Mood Change, Sweating, Anxiety, Not Thinking Clearly, Feeling Restless (circle any that apply)
Other _____ |

Evaluate your sleep last night.
Scale : 0 1 2 3 4 5 (poor 0 to excellent 5)
Bad or disturbing dreams?_____

Dizziness? y/n _____
Falls? y/n _____
Depression? y/n _____   Alcohol? y/n
Hallucinations? y/n _____   How much?_____

Did you exercise today? y/n How Long? _____ minutes
Type of Exercise: _____

Did you eat three balanced healthy meals today?
Breakfast y/n _____
Lunch y/n _____
Dinner y/n _____

What did you accomplish today? _____
_____

Date:_____   **Daily Log**   Overall Rating: 😊 😐 ☹️

Did you remember to take your medications today?	Off times: Time of day symptoms started: _____
_____am/pm y/n _____am/pm y/n _____am/pm y/n _____am/pm y/n _____am/pm y/n	Symptoms: Fatigue, Tremors, Mood Change, Sweating, Anxiety, Not Thinking Clearly, Feeling Restless (circle any that apply) Other _____

Evaluate your sleep last night.
Scale : 0 1 2 3 4 5 (poor 0 to excellent 5)
Bad or disturbing dreams?_____

Dizziness? y/n _____
Falls? y/n _____
Depression? y/n _____   Alcohol? y/n
Hallucinations? y/n _____   How much?_____

Did you exercise today? y/n How Long? _____ minutes
Type of Exercise: _____

Did you eat three balanced healthy meals today?
Breakfast y/n _____
Lunch y/n _____
Dinner y/n _____

What did you accomplish today? _____
_____

Date:_____ **Daily Log** Overall Rating: 😊 😐 ☹

Did you remember to take your medications today?	Off times: Time of day symptoms started: _____
_____am/pm y/n _____am/pm y/n _____am/pm y/n _____am/pm y/n _____am/pm y/n	Symptoms: Fatigue, Tremors, Mood Change, Sweating, Anxiety, Not Thinking Clearly, Feeling Restless (circle any that apply) Other _____

Evaluate your sleep last night.
Scale : 0 1 2 3 4 5 (poor 0 to excellent 5)
Bad or disturbing dreams?_____

Dizziness? y/n _____
Falls? y/n _____
Depression? y/n _____   Alcohol? y/n
Hallucinations? y/n _____   How much?_____

Did you exercise today? y/n How Long? _____ minutes
Type of Exercise: _____

Did you eat three balanced healthy meals today?
Breakfast y/n _____
Lunch y/n _____
Dinner y/n _____

What did you accomplish today? _____
_____

Date:_____   **Daily Log**   Overall Rating: ☺ 😐 ☹

| Did you remember to take your medications today?

_____am/pm y/n
_____am/pm y/n
_____am/pm y/n
_____am/pm y/n
_____am/pm y/n | Off times: Time of day symptoms started: _____

Symptoms: Fatigue, Tremors, Mood Change, Sweating, Anxiety, Not Thinking Clearly, Feeling Restless (circle any that apply)
Other _____ |

Evaluate your sleep last night.
Scale : 0 1 2 3 4 5 (poor 0 to excellent 5)
Bad or disturbing dreams?_____

Dizziness? y/n _____
Falls? y/n _____
Depression? y/n _____   Alcohol? y/n
Hallucinations? y/n _____   How much?_____

Did you exercise today? y/n How Long? _____ minutes
Type of Exercise: _____

Did you eat three balanced healthy meals today?
Breakfast y/n _____
Lunch y/n _____
Dinner y/n _____

What did you accomplish today? _____
_____

Date:_____ **Daily Log** Overall Rating: 😊 😐 ☹

Did you remember to take your medications today?

_____am/pm y/n
_____am/pm y/n
_____am/pm y/n
_____am/pm y/n
_____am/pm y/n

Off times: Time of day symptoms started: _____

Symptoms: Fatigue, Tremors, Mood Change, Sweating, Anxiety, Not Thinking Clearly, Feeling Restless (circle any that apply)
Other _____

Evaluate your sleep last night.
Scale : 0 1 2 3 4 5   (poor 0 to excellent 5)
Bad or disturbing dreams?_____

Dizziness? y/n _____
Falls? y/n _____
Depression? y/n _____   Alcohol? y/n
Hallucinations? y/n _____   How much?_____

Did you exercise today? y/n How Long? _____ minutes
Type of Exercise: _____

Did you eat three balanced healthy meals today?
Breakfast y/n _____
Lunch y/n _____
Dinner y/n _____

What did you accomplish today? _____
_____

Date:_____ **Daily Log** Overall Rating: 😀 😐 ☹

| Did you remember to take your medications today? _____am/pm y/n _____am/pm y/n _____am/pm y/n _____am/pm y/n _____am/pm y/n | Off times: Time of day symptoms started: _____ Symptoms: Fatigue, Tremors, Mood Change, Sweating, Anxiety, Not Thinking Clearly, Feeling Restless (circle any that apply) Other _____ |

Evaluate your sleep last night.
Scale : 0 1 2 3 4 5 (poor 0 to excellent 5)
Bad or disturbing dreams?_____

Dizziness? y/n _____
Falls? y/n _____
Depression? y/n _____   Alcohol? y/n
Hallucinations? y/n _____   How much?_____

Did you exercise today? y/n How Long? _____ minutes
Type of Exercise: _____

Did you eat three balanced healthy meals today?
Breakfast y/n _____
Lunch y/n _____
Dinner y/n _____

What did you accomplish today? _____
_____
_____

Date:_____ **Daily Log**   Overall Rating: ☺ 😐 ☹

| Did you remember to take your medications today?

_____am/pm y/n
_____am/pm y/n
_____am/pm y/n
_____am/pm y/n
_____am/pm y/n | Off times: Time of day symptoms started: _____

Symptoms: Fatigue, Tremors, Mood Change, Sweating, Anxiety, Not Thinking Clearly, Feeling Restless (circle any that apply)
Other _____ |

Evaluate your sleep last night.
Scale : 0 1 2 3 4 5 (poor 0 to excellent 5)
Bad or disturbing dreams?_____

Dizziness? y/n _____
Falls? y/n _____
Depression? y/n _____   Alcohol? y/n
Hallucinations? y/n _____   How much?_____

Did you exercise today? y/n How Long? _____ minutes
Type of Exercise: _____

Did you eat three balanced healthy meals today?
Breakfast y/n _____
Lunch y/n _____
Dinner y/n _____

What did you accomplish today? _____
_____

Date:_____ **Daily Log** Overall Rating: 😊 😐 ☹

| Did you remember to take your medications today?

_____am/pm y/n
_____am/pm y/n
_____am/pm y/n
_____am/pm y/n
_____am/pm y/n | Off times: Time of day symptoms started: _____

Symptoms: Fatigue, Tremors, Mood Change, Sweating, Anxiety, Not Thinking Clearly, Feeling Restless (circle any that apply)
Other _____ |

Evaluate your sleep last night.
Scale : 0 1 2 3 4 5 (poor 0 to excellent 5)
Bad or disturbing dreams?_____

Dizziness? y/n _____
Falls? y/n _____
Depression? y/n _____   Alcohol? y/n
Hallucinations? y/n _____   How much?_____

Did you exercise today? y/n How Long? _____ minutes
Type of Exercise: _____

Did you eat three balanced healthy meals today?
Breakfast y/n _____
Lunch y/n _____
Dinner y/n _____

What did you accomplish today? _____
_____

Date:_____ **Daily Log**   Overall Rating: ☺ 😐 ☹

| Did you remember to take your medications today?

_____am/pm y/n
_____am/pm y/n
_____am/pm y/n
_____am/pm y/n
_____am/pm y/n | Off times: Time of day symptoms started: _____

Symptoms: Fatigue, Tremors, Mood Change, Sweating, Anxiety, Not Thinking Clearly, Feeling Restless (circle any that apply)
Other _____ |

Evaluate your sleep last night.
Scale : 0 1 2 3 4 5   (poor 0 to excellent 5)
Bad or disturbing dreams?_____

Dizziness? y/n _____
Falls? y/n _____
Depression? y/n _____   Alcohol? y/n
Hallucinations? y/n _____   How much?_____

Did you exercise today? y/n How Long? _____ minutes
Type of Exercise: _____

Did you eat three balanced healthy meals today?
Breakfast y/n _____
Lunch y/n _____
Dinner y/n _____

What did you accomplish today? _____
_____

Date:_____   **Daily Log**   Overall Rating: ☺ 😐 ☹

| Did you remember to take your medications today?

_____am/pm y/n
_____am/pm y/n
_____am/pm y/n
_____am/pm y/n
_____am/pm y/n | Off times: Time of day symptoms started: _____

Symptoms: Fatigue, Tremors, Mood Change, Sweating, Anxiety, Not Thinking Clearly, Feeling Restless (circle any that apply)
Other _____ |

Evaluate your sleep last night.
Scale : 0 1 2 3 4 5 (poor 0 to excellent 5)
Bad or disturbing dreams?_____

Dizziness? y/n _____
Falls? y/n _____
Depression? y/n _____   Alcohol? y/n
Hallucinations? y/n _____   How much?_____

Did you exercise today? y/n How Long? _____ minutes
Type of Exercise: _____

Did you eat three balanced healthy meals today?
Breakfast y/n _____
Lunch y/n _____
Dinner y/n _____

What did you accomplish today? _____
_____

Date:_____ **Daily Log** Overall Rating: ☺ 😐 ☹

| Did you remember to take your medications today?

_____am/pm y/n
_____am/pm y/n
_____am/pm y/n
_____am/pm y/n
_____am/pm y/n | Off times: Time of day symptoms started: _____

Symptoms: Fatigue, Tremors, Mood Change, Sweating, Anxiety, Not Thinking Clearly, Feeling Restless (circle any that apply)
Other _____ |

Evaluate your sleep last night.
Scale : 0 1 2 3 4 5 (poor 0 to excellent 5)
Bad or disturbing dreams?_____

Dizziness? y/n _____
Falls? y/n _____
Depression? y/n _____   Alcohol? y/n
Hallucinations? y/n _____   How much?_____

Did you exercise today? y/n How Long? _____ minutes
Type of Exercise: _____

Did you eat three balanced healthy meals today?
Breakfast y/n _____
Lunch y/n _____
Dinner y/n _____

What did you accomplish today? _____
_____

Date:_____ **Daily Log** Overall Rating: ☺ 😐 ☹

Did you remember to take your medications today?

_____am/pm y/n
_____am/pm y/n
_____am/pm y/n
_____am/pm y/n
_____am/pm y/n

Off times: Time of day symptoms started: _____

Symptoms: Fatigue, Tremors, Mood Change, Sweating, Anxiety, Not Thinking Clearly, Feeling Restless (circle any that apply)
Other _____

Evaluate your sleep last night.
Scale : 0 1 2 3 4 5 (poor 0 to excellent 5)
Bad or disturbing dreams?_____

Dizziness? y/n _____
Falls? y/n _____
Depression? y/n _____   Alcohol? y/n
Hallucinations? y/n _____   How much?_____

Did you exercise today? y/n How Long? _____ minutes
Type of Exercise: _____

Did you eat three balanced healthy meals today?
Breakfast y/n _____
Lunch y/n _____
Dinner y/n _____

What did you accomplish today? _____
_____

Date:_____ **Daily Log** Overall Rating: ☺ 😐 ☹

Did you remember to take your medications today?

_____am/pm y/n
_____am/pm y/n
_____am/pm y/n
_____am/pm y/n
_____am/pm y/n

Off times: Time of day symptoms started: _____

Symptoms: Fatigue, Tremors, Mood Change, Sweating, Anxiety, Not Thinking Clearly, Feeling Restless (circle any that apply)
Other _____

Evaluate your sleep last night.
Scale : 0 1 2 3 4 5 (poor 0 to excellent 5)
Bad or disturbing dreams?_____

Dizziness? y/n _____
Falls? y/n _____
Depression? y/n _____   Alcohol? y/n
Hallucinations? y/n _____   How much?_____

Did you exercise today? y/n How Long? _____ minutes
Type of Exercise: _____

Did you eat three balanced healthy meals today?
Breakfast y/n _____
Lunch y/n _____
Dinner y/n _____

What did you accomplish today? _____
_____

Date:_____   **Daily Log**   Overall Rating: 😊 😐 ☹️

Did you remember to take your medications today?

_____am/pm y/n
_____am/pm y/n
_____am/pm y/n
_____am/pm y/n
_____am/pm y/n

Off times: Time of day symptoms started: _____

Symptoms: Fatigue, Tremors, Mood Change, Sweating, Anxiety, Not Thinking Clearly, Feeling Restless (circle any that apply)
Other _____

Evaluate your sleep last night.
Scale : 0 1 2 3 4 5 (poor 0 to excellent 5)
Bad or disturbing dreams?_____

Dizziness? y/n _____
Falls? y/n _____
Depression? y/n _____   Alcohol? y/n
Hallucinations? y/n _____   How much?_____

Did you exercise today? y/n How Long? _____ minutes
Type of Exercise: _____

Did you eat three balanced healthy meals today?
Breakfast y/n _____
Lunch y/n _____
Dinner y/n _____

What did you accomplish today? _____
_____

Date:_____ **Daily Log** Overall Rating: 😊 😐 ☹

| Did you remember to take your medications today?

_____am/pm y/n
_____am/pm y/n
_____am/pm y/n
_____am/pm y/n
_____am/pm y/n | Off times: Time of day symptoms started: _____

Symptoms: Fatigue, Tremors, Mood Change, Sweating, Anxiety, Not Thinking Clearly, Feeling Restless (circle any that apply)
Other _____ |

Evaluate your sleep last night.
Scale : 0 1 2 3 4 5   (poor 0 to excellent 5)
Bad or disturbing dreams?_____

Dizziness? y/n _____
Falls? y/n _____
Depression? y/n _____   Alcohol? y/n
Hallucinations? y/n _____   How much?_____

Did you exercise today? y/n How Long? _____ minutes
Type of Exercise: _____

Did you eat three balanced healthy meals today?
Breakfast y/n _____
Lunch y/n _____
Dinner y/n _____

What did you accomplish today? _____
_____

Date:_____   **Daily Log**   Overall Rating: 😊 😐 ☹

Did you remember to take your medications today?	Off times: Time of day symptoms started: _____
_____am/pm y/n _____am/pm y/n _____am/pm y/n _____am/pm y/n _____am/pm y/n	Symptoms: Fatigue, Tremors, Mood Change, Sweating, Anxiety, Not Thinking Clearly, Feeling Restless (circle any that apply) Other _____

Evaluate your sleep last night.
Scale : 0 1 2 3 4 5   (poor 0 to excellent 5)
Bad or disturbing dreams?_____

Dizziness? y/n _____
Falls? y/n _____
Depression? y/n _____   Alcohol? y/n
Hallucinations? y/n _____   How much?_____

Did you exercise today? y/n How Long? _____ minutes
Type of Exercise: _____

Did you eat three balanced healthy meals today?
Breakfast y/n _____
Lunch y/n _____
Dinner y/n _____

What did you accomplish today? _____
_____

Date:_____ **Daily Log** Overall Rating: 😊 😐 ☹️

| Did you remember to take your medications today?

_____am/pm y/n
_____am/pm y/n
_____am/pm y/n
_____am/pm y/n
_____am/pm y/n | Off times: Time of day symptoms started: _____

Symptoms: Fatigue, Tremors, Mood Change, Sweating, Anxiety, Not Thinking Clearly, Feeling Restless (circle any that apply)
Other _____ |

Evaluate your sleep last night.
Scale : 0 1 2 3 4 5 (poor 0 to excellent 5)
Bad or disturbing dreams?_____

Dizziness? y/n _____
Falls? y/n _____
Depression? y/n _____   Alcohol? y/n
Hallucinations? y/n _____ How much?_____

Did you exercise today? y/n How Long? _____ minutes
Type of Exercise: _____

Did you eat three balanced healthy meals today?
Breakfast y/n _____
Lunch y/n _____
Dinner y/n _____

What did you accomplish today? _____
_____

Date:_____   **Daily Log**   Overall Rating: ☺ 😐 ☹

| Did you remember to take your medications today?

_____am/pm y/n
_____am/pm y/n
_____am/pm y/n
_____am/pm y/n
_____am/pm y/n | Off times: Time of day symptoms started: _____

Symptoms: Fatigue, Tremors, Mood Change, Sweating, Anxiety, Not Thinking Clearly, Feeling Restless (circle any that apply)
Other _____ |

Evaluate your sleep last night.
Scale : 0 1 2 3 4 5 (poor 0 to excellent 5)
Bad or disturbing dreams?_____

Dizziness? y/n _____
Falls? y/n _____
Depression? y/n _____   Alcohol? y/n
Hallucinations? y/n _____   How much?_____

Did you exercise today? y/n How Long? _____ minutes
Type of Exercise: _____

Did you eat three balanced healthy meals today?
Breakfast y/n _____
Lunch y/n _____
Dinner y/n _____

What did you accomplish today? _____
_____

Date:_____ **Daily Log** Overall Rating: 😊 😐 ☹

| Did you remember to take your medications today?

_____am/pm y/n
_____am/pm y/n
_____am/pm y/n
_____am/pm y/n
_____am/pm y/n | Off times: Time of day symptoms started: _____

Symptoms: Fatigue, Tremors, Mood Change, Sweating, Anxiety, Not Thinking Clearly, Feeling Restless (circle any that apply)
Other _____ |

Evaluate your sleep last night.
Scale : 0 1 2 3 4 5 (poor 0 to excellent 5)
Bad or disturbing dreams?_____

Dizziness? y/n _____
Falls? y/n _____
Depression? y/n _____   Alcohol? y/n
Hallucinations? y/n _____   How much?_____

Did you exercise today? y/n How Long? _____ minutes
Type of Exercise: _____

Did you eat three balanced healthy meals today?
Breakfast y/n _____
Lunch y/n _____
Dinner y/n _____

What did you accomplish today? _____
_____

Date:_____ **Daily Log** Overall Rating: 😊 😐 ☹️

| Did you remember to take your medications today?

_____am/pm y/n
_____am/pm y/n
_____am/pm y/n
_____am/pm y/n
_____am/pm y/n | Off times: Time of day symptoms started: _____

Symptoms: Fatigue, Tremors, Mood Change, Sweating, Anxiety, Not Thinking Clearly, Feeling Restless (circle any that apply)
Other _____ |

Evaluate your sleep last night.
Scale : 0 1 2 3 4 5 (poor 0 to excellent 5)
Bad or disturbing dreams?_____

Dizziness? y/n _____
Falls? y/n _____
Depression? y/n _____   Alcohol? y/n
Hallucinations? y/n _____   How much?_____

Did you exercise today? y/n How Long? _____ minutes
Type of Exercise: _____

Did you eat three balanced healthy meals today?
Breakfast y/n _____
Lunch y/n _____
Dinner y/n _____

What did you accomplish today? _____
_____

Date:_____ **Daily Log** Overall Rating: 😊 😐 ☹

| Did you remember to take your medications today?

_____am/pm y/n
_____am/pm y/n
_____am/pm y/n
_____am/pm y/n
_____am/pm y/n | Off times: Time of day symptoms started: _____

Symptoms: Fatigue, Tremors, Mood Change, Sweating, Anxiety, Not Thinking Clearly, Feeling Restless (circle any that apply)
Other _____ |

Evaluate your sleep last night.
Scale : 0 1 2 3 4 5 (poor 0 to excellent 5)
Bad or disturbing dreams?_____

Dizziness? y/n _____
Falls? y/n _____
Depression? y/n _____   Alcohol? y/n
Hallucinations? y/n _____   How much?_____

Did you exercise today? y/n How Long? _____ minutes
Type of Exercise: _____

Did you eat three balanced healthy meals today?
Breakfast y/n _____
Lunch y/n _____
Dinner y/n _____

What did you accomplish today? _____
_____

Date:_____ **Daily Log** Overall Rating: 😊 😐 ☹

| Did you remember to take your medications today?

_____am/pm y/n
_____am/pm y/n
_____am/pm y/n
_____am/pm y/n
_____am/pm y/n | Off times: Time of day symptoms started: _____

Symptoms: Fatigue, Tremors, Mood Change, Sweating, Anxiety, Not Thinking Clearly, Feeling Restless (circle any that apply)
Other _____ |

Evaluate your sleep last night.
Scale : 0 1 2 3 4 5 (poor 0 to excellent 5)
Bad or disturbing dreams?_____

Dizziness? y/n _____
Falls? y/n _____
Depression? y/n _____   Alcohol? y/n
Hallucinations? y/n _____   How much?_____

Did you exercise today? y/n How Long? _____ minutes
Type of Exercise: _____

Did you eat three balanced healthy meals today?
Breakfast y/n _____
Lunch y/n _____
Dinner y/n _____

What did you accomplish today? _____
_____

Date:_____ **Daily Log** Overall Rating: 😊 😐 ☹

| Did you remember to take your medications today?

_____am/pm y/n
_____am/pm y/n
_____am/pm y/n
_____am/pm y/n
_____am/pm y/n | Off times: Time of day symptoms started: _____

Symptoms: Fatigue, Tremors, Mood Change, Sweating, Anxiety, Not Thinking Clearly, Feeling Restless (circle any that apply)
Other _____ |

Evaluate your sleep last night.
Scale : 0 1 2 3 4 5 (poor 0 to excellent 5)
Bad or disturbing dreams?_____

Dizziness? y/n _____
Falls? y/n _____
Depression? y/n _____   Alcohol? y/n
Hallucinations? y/n _____   How much?_____

Did you exercise today? y/n How Long? _____ minutes
Type of Exercise: _____

Did you eat three balanced healthy meals today?
Breakfast y/n _____
Lunch y/n _____
Dinner y/n _____

What did you accomplish today? _____
_____

Date:_____ **Daily Log** Overall Rating: 😊 😐 ☹

| Did you remember to take your medications today?

_____am/pm y/n
_____am/pm y/n
_____am/pm y/n
_____am/pm y/n
_____am/pm y/n | Off times: Time of day symptoms started: _____

Symptoms: Fatigue, Tremors, Mood Change, Sweating, Anxiety, Not Thinking Clearly, Feeling Restless (circle any that apply)
Other _____ |

Evaluate your sleep last night.
Scale : 0 1 2 3 4 5 (poor 0 to excellent 5)
Bad or disturbing dreams?_____

Dizziness? y/n _____
Falls? y/n _____
Depression? y/n _____ Alcohol? y/n
Hallucinations? y/n _____ How much?_____

Did you exercise today? y/n How Long? _____ minutes
Type of Exercise: _____

Did you eat three balanced healthy meals today?
Breakfast y/n _____
Lunch y/n _____
Dinner y/n _____

What did you accomplish today? _____
_____

Date:_____ **Daily Log** Overall Rating: 😊 😐 ☹

| Did you remember to take your medications today?

_____am/pm y/n
_____am/pm y/n
_____am/pm y/n
_____am/pm y/n
_____am/pm y/n | Off times: Time of day symptoms started: _____

Symptoms: Fatigue, Tremors, Mood Change, Sweating, Anxiety, Not Thinking Clearly, Feeling Restless (circle any that apply)
Other _____ |

Evaluate your sleep last night.
Scale : 0 1 2 3 4 5   (poor 0 to excellent 5)
Bad or disturbing dreams?_____

Dizziness? y/n _____
Falls? y/n _____
Depression? y/n _____   Alcohol? y/n
Hallucinations? y/n _____   How much?_____

Did you exercise today? y/n How Long? _____ minutes
Type of Exercise: _____

Did you eat three balanced healthy meals today?
Breakfast y/n _____
Lunch y/n _____
Dinner y/n _____

What did you accomplish today? _____
_____

Date:_____ **Daily Log** Overall Rating: 😊 😐 ☹

Did you remember to take your medications today?	Off times: Time of day symptoms started: _____
_____am/pm y/n _____am/pm y/n _____am/pm y/n _____am/pm y/n _____am/pm y/n	Symptoms: Fatigue, Tremors, Mood Change, Sweating, Anxiety, Not Thinking Clearly, Feeling Restless (circle any that apply) Other _____

Evaluate your sleep last night.
Scale : 0 1 2 3 4 5 (poor 0 to excellent 5)
Bad or disturbing dreams?_____

Dizziness? y/n _____
Falls? y/n _____
Depression? y/n _____   Alcohol? y/n
Hallucinations? y/n _____   How much?_____

Did you exercise today? y/n How Long? _____ minutes
Type of Exercise: _____

Did you eat three balanced healthy meals today?
Breakfast y/n _____
Lunch y/n _____
Dinner y/n _____

What did you accomplish today? _____
_____

Date:_____   **Daily Log**   Overall Rating: ☺ 😐 ☹

| Did you remember to take your medications today?

_____am/pm y/n
_____am/pm y/n
_____am/pm y/n
_____am/pm y/n
_____am/pm y/n | Off times: Time of day symptoms started: _____

Symptoms: Fatigue, Tremors, Mood Change, Sweating, Anxiety, Not Thinking Clearly, Feeling Restless (circle any that apply)
Other _____ |

Evaluate your sleep last night.
Scale : 0 1 2 3 4 5 (poor 0 to excellent 5)
Bad or disturbing dreams?_____

Dizziness? y/n _____
Falls? y/n _____
Depression? y/n _____   Alcohol? y/n
Hallucinations? y/n _____   How much?_____

Did you exercise today? y/n How Long? _____ minutes
Type of Exercise: _____

Did you eat three balanced healthy meals today?
Breakfast y/n _____
Lunch y/n _____
Dinner y/n _____

What did you accomplish today? _____
_____

Date:_____   **Daily Log**   Overall Rating: 😊 😐 ☹

Did you remember to take your medications today? _____am/pm y/n _____am/pm y/n _____am/pm y/n _____am/pm y/n _____am/pm y/n	Off times: Time of day symptoms started: _____ Symptoms: Fatigue, Tremors, Mood Change, Sweating, Anxiety, Not Thinking Clearly, Feeling Restless (circle any that apply) Other _____

Evaluate your sleep last night.
Scale : 0 1 2 3 4 5 (poor 0 to excellent 5)
Bad or disturbing dreams?_____

Dizziness? y/n _____
Falls? y/n _____
Depression? y/n _____   Alcohol? y/n
Hallucinations? y/n _____   How much?_____

Did you exercise today? y/n How Long? _____ minutes
Type of Exercise: _____

Did you eat three balanced healthy meals today?
Breakfast y/n _____
Lunch y/n _____
Dinner y/n _____

What did you accomplish today? _____
_____

Date:_____ **Daily Log** Overall Rating: 😊 😐 ☹

| Did you remember to take your medications today?

_____am/pm y/n
_____am/pm y/n
_____am/pm y/n
_____am/pm y/n
_____am/pm y/n | Off times: Time of day symptoms started: _____

Symptoms: Fatigue, Tremors, Mood Change, Sweating, Anxiety, Not Thinking Clearly, Feeling Restless (circle any that apply)
Other _____ |

Evaluate your sleep last night.
Scale : 0 1 2 3 4 5 (poor 0 to excellent 5)
Bad or disturbing dreams?_____

Dizziness? y/n _____
Falls? y/n _____
Depression? y/n _____ Alcohol? y/n
Hallucinations? y/n _____ How much?_____

Did you exercise today? y/n How Long? _____ minutes
Type of Exercise: _____

Did you eat three balanced healthy meals today?
Breakfast y/n _____
Lunch y/n _____
Dinner y/n _____

What did you accomplish today? _____
_____

Date:_____   **Daily Log**   Overall Rating: 😊 😐 ☹

Did you remember to take your medications today?

_____am/pm y/n
_____am/pm y/n
_____am/pm y/n
_____am/pm y/n
_____am/pm y/n

Off times: Time of day symptoms started: _____

Symptoms: Fatigue, Tremors, Mood Change, Sweating, Anxiety, Not Thinking Clearly, Feeling Restless (circle any that apply)
Other _____

Evaluate your sleep last night.
Scale : 0 1 2 3 4 5 (poor 0 to excellent 5)
Bad or disturbing dreams?_____

Dizziness? y/n _____
Falls? y/n _____
Depression? y/n _____   Alcohol? y/n
Hallucinations? y/n _____   How much?_____

Did you exercise today? y/n How Long? _____ minutes
Type of Exercise: _____

Did you eat three balanced healthy meals today?
Breakfast y/n _____
Lunch y/n _____
Dinner y/n _____

What did you accomplish today? _____
_____

Date:_____ **Daily Log**   Overall Rating: ☺ 😐 ☹

| Did you remember to take your medications today?

_____am/pm y/n
_____am/pm y/n
_____am/pm y/n
_____am/pm y/n
_____am/pm y/n | Off times: Time of day symptoms started: _____

Symptoms: Fatigue, Tremors, Mood Change, Sweating, Anxiety, Not Thinking Clearly, Feeling Restless (circle any that apply)
Other _____ |

Evaluate your sleep last night.
Scale : 0 1 2 3 4 5 (poor 0 to excellent 5)
Bad or disturbing dreams?_____

Dizziness? y/n _____
Falls? y/n _____
Depression? y/n _____   Alcohol? y/n
Hallucinations? y/n _____   How much?_____

Did you exercise today? y/n How Long? _____ minutes
Type of Exercise: _____

Did you eat three balanced healthy meals today?
Breakfast y/n _____
Lunch y/n _____
Dinner y/n _____

What did you accomplish today? _____
_____

Date:_____ **Daily Log** Overall Rating: 😊 😐 ☹

Did you remember to take your medications today?	Off times: Time of day symptoms started: _____
_____am/pm y/n _____am/pm y/n _____am/pm y/n _____am/pm y/n _____am/pm y/n	Symptoms: Fatigue, Tremors, Mood Change, Sweating, Anxiety, Not Thinking Clearly, Feeling Restless (circle any that apply) Other _____

Evaluate your sleep last night.
Scale : 0 1 2 3 4 5 (poor 0 to excellent 5)
Bad or disturbing dreams?_____

Dizziness? y/n _____
Falls? y/n _____
Depression? y/n _____   Alcohol? y/n
Hallucinations? y/n _____   How much?_____

Did you exercise today? y/n How Long? _____ minutes
Type of Exercise: _____

Did you eat three balanced healthy meals today?
Breakfast y/n _____
Lunch y/n _____
Dinner y/n _____

What did you accomplish today? _____
_____

Date:_____ **Daily Log** Overall Rating: ☺ 😐 ☹

Did you remember to take your medications today?	Off times: Time of day symptoms started: _____
_____am/pm y/n _____am/pm y/n _____am/pm y/n _____am/pm y/n _____am/pm y/n	Symptoms: Fatigue, Tremors, Mood Change, Sweating, Anxiety, Not Thinking Clearly, Feeling Restless (circle any that apply) Other _____

Evaluate your sleep last night.
Scale : 0 1 2 3 4 5 (poor 0 to excellent 5)
Bad or disturbing dreams?_____

Dizziness? y/n _____
Falls? y/n _____
Depression? y/n _____   Alcohol? y/n
Hallucinations? y/n _____   How much?_____

Did you exercise today? y/n How Long? _____ minutes
Type of Exercise: _____

Did you eat three balanced healthy meals today?
Breakfast y/n _____
Lunch y/n _____
Dinner y/n _____

What did you accomplish today? _____
_____

Date:_____ **Daily Log** Overall Rating: 😊 😐 ☹

| Did you remember to take your medications today?

_____am/pm y/n
_____am/pm y/n
_____am/pm y/n
_____am/pm y/n
_____am/pm y/n | Off times: Time of day symptoms started: _____

Symptoms: Fatigue, Tremors, Mood Change, Sweating, Anxiety, Not Thinking Clearly, Feeling Restless (circle any that apply)
Other _____ |

Evaluate your sleep last night.
Scale : 0 1 2 3 4 5   (poor 0 to excellent 5)
Bad or disturbing dreams?_____

Dizziness? y/n _____
Falls? y/n _____
Depression? y/n _____   Alcohol? y/n
Hallucinations? y/n _____   How much?_____

Did you exercise today? y/n How Long? _____ minutes
Type of Exercise: _____

Did you eat three balanced healthy meals today?
Breakfast y/n _____
Lunch y/n _____
Dinner y/n _____

What did you accomplish today? _____
_____

Date:_____ **Daily Log** Overall Rating: 😊 😐 ☹️

| Did you remember to take your medications today?

_____am/pm y/n
_____am/pm y/n
_____am/pm y/n
_____am/pm y/n
_____am/pm y/n | Off times: Time of day symptoms started: _____

Symptoms: Fatigue, Tremors, Mood Change, Sweating, Anxiety, Not Thinking Clearly, Feeling Restless (circle any that apply)
Other _____ |

Evaluate your sleep last night.
Scale : 0 1 2 3 4 5 (poor 0 to excellent 5)
Bad or disturbing dreams?_____

Dizziness? y/n _____
Falls? y/n _____
Depression? y/n _____   Alcohol? y/n
Hallucinations? y/n _____   How much?_____

Did you exercise today? y/n How Long? _____ minutes
Type of Exercise: _____

Did you eat three balanced healthy meals today?
Breakfast y/n _____
Lunch y/n _____
Dinner y/n _____

What did you accomplish today? _____
_____

Date:_____ **Daily Log** Overall Rating: 😊 😐 ☹️

Did you remember to take your medications today?	Off times: Time of day symptoms started: _____
_____am/pm y/n _____am/pm y/n _____am/pm y/n _____am/pm y/n _____am/pm y/n	Symptoms: Fatigue, Tremors, Mood Change, Sweating, Anxiety, Not Thinking Clearly, Feeling Restless (circle any that apply) Other _____

Evaluate your sleep last night.
Scale : 0 1 2 3 4 5 (poor 0 to excellent 5)
Bad or disturbing dreams?_____

Dizziness? y/n _____
Falls? y/n _____
Depression? y/n _____   Alcohol? y/n
Hallucinations? y/n _____   How much?_____

Did you exercise today? y/n How Long? _____ minutes
Type of Exercise: _____

Did you eat three balanced healthy meals today?
Breakfast y/n _____
Lunch y/n _____
Dinner y/n _____

What did you accomplish today? _____
_____

Date:_____ **Daily Log** Overall Rating: 😊 😐 ☹️

| Did you remember to take your medications today?

_____am/pm y/n
_____am/pm y/n
_____am/pm y/n
_____am/pm y/n
_____am/pm y/n | Off times: Time of day symptoms started: _____

Symptoms: Fatigue, Tremors, Mood Change, Sweating, Anxiety, Not Thinking Clearly, Feeling Restless (circle any that apply)
Other _____ |

Evaluate your sleep last night.
Scale : 0 1 2 3 4 5 (poor 0 to excellent 5)
Bad or disturbing dreams?_____

Dizziness? y/n _____
Falls? y/n _____
Depression? y/n _____   Alcohol? y/n
Hallucinations? y/n _____   How much?_____

Did you exercise today? y/n How Long? _____ minutes
Type of Exercise: _____

Did you eat three balanced healthy meals today?
Breakfast y/n _____
Lunch y/n _____
Dinner y/n _____

What did you accomplish today? _____
_____

Date:_____ **Daily Log** Overall Rating: 😊 😐 ☹️

Did you remember to take your medications today?

_____am/pm y/n
_____am/pm y/n
_____am/pm y/n
_____am/pm y/n
_____am/pm y/n

Off times: Time of day symptoms started: _____

Symptoms: Fatigue, Tremors, Mood Change, Sweating, Anxiety, Not Thinking Clearly, Feeling Restless (circle any that apply)
Other _____

Evaluate your sleep last night.
Scale : 0 1 2 3 4 5   (poor 0 to excellent 5)
Bad or disturbing dreams?_____

Dizziness? y/n _____
Falls? y/n _____
Depression? y/n _____   Alcohol? y/n
Hallucinations? y/n _____   How much?_____

Did you exercise today? y/n How Long? _____ minutes
Type of Exercise: _____

Did you eat three balanced healthy meals today?
Breakfast y/n _____
Lunch y/n _____
Dinner y/n _____

What did you accomplish today? _____
_____

Date:_____   **Daily Log**   Overall Rating: 😊 😐 ☹

| Did you remember to take your medications today?

_____am/pm y/n
_____am/pm y/n
_____am/pm y/n
_____am/pm y/n
_____am/pm y/n | Off times: Time of day symptoms started: _____

Symptoms: Fatigue, Tremors, Mood Change, Sweating, Anxiety, Not Thinking Clearly, Feeling Restless (circle any that apply)
Other _____ |

Evaluate your sleep last night.
Scale : 0 1 2 3 4 5   (poor 0 to excellent 5)
Bad or disturbing dreams?_____

Dizziness? y/n _____
Falls? y/n _____
Depression? y/n _____   Alcohol? y/n
Hallucinations? y/n _____   How much?_____

Did you exercise today? y/n How Long? _____ minutes
Type of Exercise: _____

Did you eat three balanced healthy meals today?
Breakfast y/n _____
Lunch y/n _____
Dinner y/n _____

What did you accomplish today? _____
_____

Date:_____   **Daily Log**   Overall Rating: 🙂 😐 ☹

Did you remember to take your medications today?	Off times: Time of day symptoms started: _____
_____am/pm y/n _____am/pm y/n _____am/pm y/n _____am/pm y/n _____am/pm y/n	Symptoms: Fatigue, Tremors, Mood Change, Sweating, Anxiety, Not Thinking Clearly, Feeling Restless (circle any that apply) Other _____

Evaluate your sleep last night.
Scale : 0 1 2 3 4 5   (poor 0 to excellent 5)
Bad or disturbing dreams?_____

Dizziness? y/n _____
Falls? y/n _____
Depression? y/n _____   Alcohol? y/n
Hallucinations? y/n _____   How much?_____

Did you exercise today? y/n How Long? _____ minutes
Type of Exercise: _____

Did you eat three balanced healthy meals today?
Breakfast y/n _____
Lunch y/n _____
Dinner y/n _____

What did you accomplish today? _____
_____

Date:_____ **Daily Log** Overall Rating: 😊 😐 ☹

Did you remember to take your medications today?	Off times: Time of day symptoms started: _____
_____am/pm y/n _____am/pm y/n _____am/pm y/n _____am/pm y/n _____am/pm y/n	Symptoms: Fatigue, Tremors, Mood Change, Sweating, Anxiety, Not Thinking Clearly, Feeling Restless (circle any that apply) Other _____

Evaluate your sleep last night.
Scale : 0 1 2 3 4 5 (poor 0 to excellent 5)
Bad or disturbing dreams?_____

Dizziness? y/n _____
Falls? y/n _____
Depression? y/n _____   Alcohol? y/n
Hallucinations? y/n _____   How much?_____

Did you exercise today? y/n How Long? _____ minutes
Type of Exercise: _____

Did you eat three balanced healthy meals today?
Breakfast y/n _____
Lunch y/n _____
Dinner y/n _____

What did you accomplish today? _____
_____

Date:_____ **Daily Log** Overall Rating: 😊 😐 ☹

Did you remember to take your medications today?

_____am/pm y/n
_____am/pm y/n
_____am/pm y/n
_____am/pm y/n
_____am/pm y/n

Off times: Time of day symptoms started: _____

Symptoms: Fatigue, Tremors, Mood Change, Sweating, Anxiety, Not Thinking Clearly, Feeling Restless (circle any that apply)
Other _____

Evaluate your sleep last night.
Scale : 0 1 2 3 4 5   (poor 0 to excellent 5)
Bad or disturbing dreams?_____

Dizziness? y/n _____
Falls? y/n _____
Depression? y/n _____
Hallucinations? y/n _____

Alcohol? y/n
How much?_____

Did you exercise today? y/n How Long? _____ minutes
Type of Exercise: _____

Did you eat three balanced healthy meals today?
Breakfast y/n _____
Lunch y/n _____
Dinner y/n _____

What did you accomplish today? _____
_____

Date:_____ **Daily Log** Overall Rating: 😃 😐 ☹️

| Did you remember to take your medications today?

_____am/pm y/n
_____am/pm y/n
_____am/pm y/n
_____am/pm y/n
_____am/pm y/n | Off times: Time of day symptoms started: _____

Symptoms: Fatigue, Tremors, Mood Change, Sweating, Anxiety, Not Thinking Clearly, Feeling Restless (circle any that apply)
Other _____ |

Evaluate your sleep last night.
Scale : 0 1 2 3 4 5 (poor 0 to excellent 5)
Bad or disturbing dreams?_____

Dizziness? y/n _____
Falls? y/n _____
Depression? y/n _____   Alcohol? y/n
Hallucinations? y/n _____   How much?_____

Did you exercise today? y/n How Long? _____ minutes
Type of Exercise: _____

Did you eat three balanced healthy meals today?
Breakfast y/n _____
Lunch y/n _____
Dinner y/n _____

What did you accomplish today? _____
_____

Date:_____   **Daily Log**   Overall Rating: 😊 😐 ☹

| Did you remember to take your medications today?

_____am/pm y/n
_____am/pm y/n
_____am/pm y/n
_____am/pm y/n
_____am/pm y/n | Off times: Time of day symptoms started: _____

Symptoms: Fatigue, Tremors, Mood Change, Sweating, Anxiety, Not Thinking Clearly, Feeling Restless (circle any that apply)
Other _____ |

Evaluate your sleep last night.
Scale : 0 1 2 3 4 5 (poor 0 to excellent 5)
Bad or disturbing dreams?_____

Dizziness? y/n _____
Falls? y/n _____
Depression? y/n _____   Alcohol? y/n
Hallucinations? y/n _____   How much?_____

Did you exercise today? y/n How Long? _____ minutes
Type of Exercise: _____

Did you eat three balanced healthy meals today?
Breakfast y/n _____
Lunch y/n _____
Dinner y/n _____

What did you accomplish today? _____
_____

Date:_____ **Daily Log** Overall Rating: ☺ 😐 ☹

Did you remember to take your medications today?

_____am/pm y/n
_____am/pm y/n
_____am/pm y/n
_____am/pm y/n
_____am/pm y/n

Off times: Time of day symptoms started: _____

Symptoms: Fatigue, Tremors, Mood Change, Sweating, Anxiety, Not Thinking Clearly, Feeling Restless (circle any that apply)
Other _____

Evaluate your sleep last night.
Scale : 0 1 2 3 4 5   (poor 0 to excellent 5)
Bad or disturbing dreams?_____

Dizziness? y/n _____
Falls? y/n _____
Depression? y/n _____   Alcohol? y/n
Hallucinations? y/n _____   How much?_____

Did you exercise today? y/n How Long? _____ minutes
Type of Exercise: _____

Did you eat three balanced healthy meals today?
Breakfast y/n _____
Lunch y/n _____
Dinner y/n _____

What did you accomplish today? _____
_____

Date:_____ **Daily Log** Overall Rating: 😊 😐 ☹

| Did you remember to take your medications today?

_____am/pm y/n
_____am/pm y/n
_____am/pm y/n
_____am/pm y/n
_____am/pm y/n | Off times: Time of day symptoms started: _____

Symptoms: Fatigue, Tremors, Mood Change, Sweating, Anxiety, Not Thinking Clearly, Feeling Restless (circle any that apply)
Other _____ |

Evaluate your sleep last night.
Scale : 0 1 2 3 4 5 (poor 0 to excellent 5)
Bad or disturbing dreams?_____

Dizziness? y/n _____
Falls? y/n _____
Depression? y/n _____   Alcohol? y/n
Hallucinations? y/n _____   How much?_____

Did you exercise today? y/n How Long? _____ minutes
Type of Exercise: _____

Did you eat three balanced healthy meals today?
Breakfast y/n _____
Lunch y/n _____
Dinner y/n _____

What did you accomplish today? _____
_____

Date:_____ **Daily Log** Overall Rating: 😊 😐 ☹

| Did you remember to take your medications today?

_____am/pm y/n
_____am/pm y/n
_____am/pm y/n
_____am/pm y/n
_____am/pm y/n | Off times: Time of day symptoms started: _____

Symptoms: Fatigue, Tremors, Mood Change, Sweating, Anxiety, Not Thinking Clearly, Feeling Restless (circle any that apply)
Other _____ |

Evaluate your sleep last night.
Scale : 0 1 2 3 4 5 (poor 0 to excellent 5)
Bad or disturbing dreams?_____

Dizziness? y/n _____
Falls? y/n _____
Depression? y/n _____   Alcohol? y/n
Hallucinations? y/n _____   How much?_____

Did you exercise today? y/n How Long? _____ minutes
Type of Exercise: _____

Did you eat three balanced healthy meals today?
Breakfast y/n _____
Lunch y/n _____
Dinner y/n _____

What did you accomplish today? _____
_____

Date:_____ **Daily Log** Overall Rating: 😊 😐 ☹

| Did you remember to take your medications today?

_____am/pm y/n
_____am/pm y/n
_____am/pm y/n
_____am/pm y/n
_____am/pm y/n | Off times: Time of day symptoms started: _____

Symptoms: Fatigue, Tremors, Mood Change, Sweating, Anxiety, Not Thinking Clearly, Feeling Restless (circle any that apply)
Other _____ |

Evaluate your sleep last night.
Scale : 0 1 2 3 4 5 (poor 0 to excellent 5)
Bad or disturbing dreams?_____

Dizziness? y/n _____
Falls? y/n _____
Depression? y/n _____   Alcohol? y/n
Hallucinations? y/n _____   How much?_____

Did you exercise today? y/n How Long? _____ minutes
Type of Exercise: _____

Did you eat three balanced healthy meals today?
Breakfast y/n _____
Lunch y/n _____
Dinner y/n _____

What did you accomplish today? _____
_____

Date:_____ **Daily Log** Overall Rating: ☺ 😐 ☹

| Did you remember to take your medications today?

 _____am/pm y/n
 _____am/pm y/n
 _____am/pm y/n
 _____am/pm y/n
 _____am/pm y/n | Off times: Time of day symptoms started: _____

 Symptoms: Fatigue, Tremors, Mood Change, Sweating, Anxiety, Not Thinking Clearly, Feeling Restless (circle any that apply)
 Other _____ |

Evaluate your sleep last night.
Scale : 0 1 2 3 4 5   (poor 0 to excellent 5)
Bad or disturbing dreams?_____

Dizziness? y/n _____
Falls? y/n _____
Depression? y/n _____   Alcohol? y/n
Hallucinations? y/n _____ How much?_____

Did you exercise today? y/n How Long? _____ minutes
Type of Exercise: _____

Did you eat three balanced healthy meals today?
Breakfast y/n _____
Lunch y/n _____
Dinner y/n _____

What did you accomplish today? _____
_____

Date:_____ **Daily Log** Overall Rating: 😊 😐 ☹

| Did you remember to take your medications today?

_____am/pm y/n
_____am/pm y/n
_____am/pm y/n
_____am/pm y/n
_____am/pm y/n | Off times: Time of day symptoms started: _____

Symptoms: Fatigue, Tremors, Mood Change, Sweating, Anxiety, Not Thinking Clearly, Feeling Restless (circle any that apply)
Other _____ |

Evaluate your sleep last night.
Scale : 0 1 2 3 4 5 (poor 0 to excellent 5)
Bad or disturbing dreams?_____

Dizziness? y/n _____
Falls? y/n _____
Depression? y/n _____   Alcohol? y/n
Hallucinations? y/n _____   How much?_____

Did you exercise today? y/n How Long? _____ minutes
Type of Exercise: _____

Did you eat three balanced healthy meals today?
Breakfast y/n _____
Lunch y/n _____
Dinner y/n _____

What did you accomplish today? _____
_____

Date:_____   **Daily Log**   Overall Rating: 😊 😐 ☹️

Did you remember to take your medications today?	Off times: Time of day symptoms started: _____
_____am/pm y/n _____am/pm y/n _____am/pm y/n _____am/pm y/n _____am/pm y/n	Symptoms: Fatigue, Tremors, Mood Change, Sweating, Anxiety, Not Thinking Clearly, Feeling Restless (circle any that apply) Other _____

Evaluate your sleep last night.
Scale : 0 1 2 3 4 5   (poor 0 to excellent 5)
Bad or disturbing dreams?_____

Dizziness? y/n _____
Falls? y/n _____
Depression? y/n _____   Alcohol? y/n
Hallucinations? y/n _____   How much?_____

Did you exercise today? y/n How Long? _____ minutes
Type of Exercise: _____

Did you eat three balanced healthy meals today?
Breakfast y/n _____
Lunch y/n _____
Dinner y/n _____

What did you accomplish today? _____
_____

Date:_____ **Daily Log** Overall Rating: 😊 😐 ☹

| Did you remember to take your medications today?

_____am/pm y/n
_____am/pm y/n
_____am/pm y/n
_____am/pm y/n
_____am/pm y/n | Off times: Time of day symptoms started: _____

Symptoms: Fatigue, Tremors, Mood Change, Sweating, Anxiety, Not Thinking Clearly, Feeling Restless (circle any that apply)
Other _____ |

Evaluate your sleep last night.
Scale : 0 1 2 3 4 5 (poor 0 to excellent 5)
Bad or disturbing dreams?_____

Dizziness? y/n _____
Falls? y/n _____
Depression? y/n _____   Alcohol? y/n
Hallucinations? y/n _____   How much?_____

Did you exercise today? y/n How Long? _____ minutes
Type of Exercise: _____

Did you eat three balanced healthy meals today?
Breakfast y/n _____
Lunch y/n _____
Dinner y/n _____

What did you accomplish today? _____
_____

Date:_____   **Daily Log**   Overall Rating: ☺ 😐 ☹

| Did you remember to take your medications today?

_____ am/pm y/n
_____ am/pm y/n
_____ am/pm y/n
_____ am/pm y/n
_____ am/pm y/n | Off times: Time of day symptoms started: _____

Symptoms: Fatigue, Tremors, Mood Change, Sweating, Anxiety, Not Thinking Clearly, Feeling Restless (circle any that apply)
Other _____ |

Evaluate your sleep last night.
Scale : 0 1 2 3 4 5   (poor 0 to excellent 5)
Bad or disturbing dreams?_____

Dizziness? y/n _____
Falls? y/n _____
Depression? y/n _____   Alcohol? y/n
Hallucinations? y/n _____   How much?_____

Did you exercise today? y/n How Long? _____ minutes
Type of Exercise: _____

Did you eat three balanced healthy meals today?
Breakfast y/n _____
Lunch y/n _____
Dinner y/n _____

What did you accomplish today? _____
_____

Date:_____ **Daily Log**   Overall Rating: 😊 😐 ☹

| Did you remember to take your medications today?

_____am/pm y/n
_____am/pm y/n
_____am/pm y/n
_____am/pm y/n
_____am/pm y/n | Off times: Time of day symptoms started: _____

Symptoms: Fatigue, Tremors, Mood Change, Sweating, Anxiety, Not Thinking Clearly, Feeling Restless (circle any that apply)
Other _____ |

Evaluate your sleep last night.
Scale : 0 1 2 3 4 5   (poor 0 to excellent 5)
Bad or disturbing dreams?_____

Dizziness? y/n _____
Falls? y/n _____
Depression? y/n _____   Alcohol? y/n
Hallucinations? y/n _____   How much?_____

Did you exercise today? y/n How Long? _____ minutes
Type of Exercise: _____

Did you eat three balanced healthy meals today?
Breakfast y/n _____
Lunch y/n _____
Dinner y/n _____

What did you accomplish today? _____
_____

Date:_____ **Daily Log** Overall Rating: 😊 😐 ☹️

| Did you remember to take your medications today?

_____am/pm y/n
_____am/pm y/n
_____am/pm y/n
_____am/pm y/n
_____am/pm y/n | Off times: Time of day symptoms started: _____

Symptoms: Fatigue, Tremors, Mood Change, Sweating, Anxiety, Not Thinking Clearly, Feeling Restless (circle any that apply)
Other _____ |

Evaluate your sleep last night.
Scale : 0 1 2 3 4 5 (poor 0 to excellent 5)
Bad or disturbing dreams?_____

Dizziness? y/n _____
Falls? y/n _____
Depression? y/n _____   Alcohol? y/n
Hallucinations? y/n _____   How much?_____

Did you exercise today? y/n How Long? _____ minutes
Type of Exercise: _____

Did you eat three balanced healthy meals today?
Breakfast y/n _____
Lunch y/n _____
Dinner y/n _____

What did you accomplish today? _____
_____

Date:_____ **Daily Log** Overall Rating: ☺ 😐 ☹

| Did you remember to take your medications today?

_____am/pm y/n
_____am/pm y/n
_____am/pm y/n
_____am/pm y/n
_____am/pm y/n | Off times: Time of day symptoms started: _____

Symptoms: Fatigue, Tremors, Mood Change, Sweating, Anxiety, Not Thinking Clearly, Feeling Restless (circle any that apply)
Other _____ |

Evaluate your sleep last night.
Scale : 0 1 2 3 4 5 (poor 0 to excellent 5)
Bad or disturbing dreams?_____

Dizziness? y/n _____
Falls? y/n _____
Depression? y/n _____   Alcohol? y/n
Hallucinations? y/n _____   How much?_____

Did you exercise today? y/n How Long? _____ minutes
Type of Exercise: _____

Did you eat three balanced healthy meals today?
Breakfast y/n _____
Lunch y/n _____
Dinner y/n _____

What did you accomplish today? _____
_____

Date:_____ **Daily Log** Overall Rating: 😊 😐 ☹️

Did you remember to take your medications today?	Off times: Time of day symptoms started: _____
_____am/pm y/n _____am/pm y/n _____am/pm y/n _____am/pm y/n _____am/pm y/n	Symptoms: Fatigue, Tremors, Mood Change, Sweating, Anxiety, Not Thinking Clearly, Feeling Restless (circle any that apply) Other _____

Evaluate your sleep last night.
Scale : 0 1 2 3 4 5   (poor 0 to excellent 5)
Bad or disturbing dreams?_____

Dizziness? y/n _____
Falls? y/n _____
Depression? y/n _____   Alcohol? y/n
Hallucinations? y/n _____   How much?_____

Did you exercise today? y/n How Long? _____ minutes
Type of Exercise: _____

Did you eat three balanced healthy meals today?
Breakfast y/n _____
Lunch y/n _____
Dinner y/n _____

What did you accomplish today? _____
_____

Date:_____   **Daily Log**   Overall Rating: 😊 😐 ☹

Did you remember to take your medications today? _____am/pm y/n _____am/pm y/n _____am/pm y/n _____am/pm y/n _____am/pm y/n	Off times: Time of day symptoms started: _____ Symptoms: Fatigue, Tremors, Mood Change, Sweating, Anxiety, Not Thinking Clearly, Feeling Restless (circle any that apply) Other _____

Evaluate your sleep last night.
Scale : 0 1 2 3 4 5   (poor 0 to excellent 5)
Bad or disturbing dreams?_____

Dizziness? y/n _____
Falls? y/n _____
Depression? y/n _____   Alcohol? y/n
Hallucinations? y/n _____   How much?_____

Did you exercise today? y/n How Long? _____ minutes
Type of Exercise: _____

Did you eat three balanced healthy meals today?
Breakfast y/n _____
Lunch y/n _____
Dinner y/n _____

What did you accomplish today? _____
_____

Date:_____ **Daily Log** Overall Rating: 😊 😐 ☹️

| Did you remember to take your medications today?

_____am/pm y/n
_____am/pm y/n
_____am/pm y/n
_____am/pm y/n
_____am/pm y/n | Off times: Time of day symptoms started: _____

Symptoms: Fatigue, Tremors, Mood Change, Sweating, Anxiety, Not Thinking Clearly, Feeling Restless (circle any that apply)
Other _____ |

Evaluate your sleep last night.
Scale : 0 1 2 3 4 5   (poor 0 to excellent 5)
Bad or disturbing dreams?_____

Dizziness? y/n _____
Falls? y/n _____
Depression? y/n _____   Alcohol? y/n
Hallucinations? y/n _____   How much?_____

Did you exercise today? y/n How Long? _____ minutes
Type of Exercise: _____

Did you eat three balanced healthy meals today?
Breakfast y/n _____
Lunch y/n _____
Dinner y/n _____

What did you accomplish today? _____
_____

Date:_____ **Daily Log** Overall Rating: 😊 😐 ☹

| Did you remember to take your medications today?

_____ am/pm y/n
_____ am/pm y/n
_____ am/pm y/n
_____ am/pm y/n
_____ am/pm y/n | Off times: Time of day symptoms started: _____

Symptoms: Fatigue, Tremors, Mood Change, Sweating, Anxiety, Not Thinking Clearly, Feeling Restless (circle any that apply)
Other _____ |

Evaluate your sleep last night.
Scale : 0 1 2 3 4 5 (poor 0 to excellent 5)
Bad or disturbing dreams?_____

Dizziness? y/n _____
Falls? y/n _____
Depression? y/n _____   Alcohol? y/n
Hallucinations? y/n _____   How much?_____

Did you exercise today? y/n How Long? _____ minutes
Type of Exercise: _____

Did you eat three balanced healthy meals today?
Breakfast y/n _____
Lunch y/n _____
Dinner y/n _____

What did you accomplish today? _____
_____

Date:_____   **Daily Log**   Overall Rating: ☺ 😐 ☹

| Did you remember to take your medications today? _____am/pm y/n _____am/pm y/n _____am/pm y/n _____am/pm y/n _____am/pm y/n | Off times: Time of day symptoms started: _____ Symptoms: Fatigue, Tremors, Mood Change, Sweating, Anxiety, Not Thinking Clearly, Feeling Restless (circle any that apply) Other _____ |

Evaluate your sleep last night.
Scale : 0 1 2 3 4 5   (poor 0 to excellent 5)
Bad or disturbing dreams?_____

Dizziness? y/n _____
Falls? y/n _____
Depression? y/n _____   Alcohol? y/n
Hallucinations? y/n _____   How much?_____

Did you exercise today? y/n   How Long? _____ minutes
Type of Exercise: _____

Did you eat three balanced healthy meals today?
Breakfast y/n _____
Lunch y/n _____
Dinner y/n _____

What did you accomplish today? _____
_____

Date:_____ **Daily Log** Overall Rating: 🙂 😐 ☹️

| Did you remember to take your medications today?

_____am/pm y/n
_____am/pm y/n
_____am/pm y/n
_____am/pm y/n
_____am/pm y/n | Off times: Time of day symptoms started: _____

Symptoms: Fatigue, Tremors, Mood Change, Sweating, Anxiety, Not Thinking Clearly, Feeling Restless (circle any that apply)
Other _____ |

Evaluate your sleep last night.
Scale : 0 1 2 3 4 5 (poor 0 to excellent 5)
Bad or disturbing dreams?_____

Dizziness? y/n _____
Falls? y/n _____
Depression? y/n _____   Alcohol? y/n
Hallucinations? y/n _____   How much?_____

Did you exercise today? y/n How Long? _____ minutes
Type of Exercise: _____

Did you eat three balanced healthy meals today?
Breakfast y/n _____
Lunch y/n _____
Dinner y/n _____

What did you accomplish today? _____
_____

Date:_____ **Daily Log** Overall Rating: 🙂 😐 ☹️

Did you remember to take your medications today?	Off times: Time of day symptoms started: _____
_____am/pm y/n _____am/pm y/n _____am/pm y/n _____am/pm y/n _____am/pm y/n	Symptoms: Fatigue, Tremors, Mood Change, Sweating, Anxiety, Not Thinking Clearly, Feeling Restless (circle any that apply) Other _____

Evaluate your sleep last night.
Scale : 0 1 2 3 4 5 (poor 0 to excellent 5)
Bad or disturbing dreams?_____

Dizziness? y/n _____
Falls? y/n _____
Depression? y/n _____ Alcohol? y/n
Hallucinations? y/n _____ How much?_____

Did you exercise today? y/n How Long? _____ minutes
Type of Exercise: _____

Did you eat three balanced healthy meals today?
Breakfast y/n _____
Lunch y/n _____
Dinner y/n _____

What did you accomplish today? _____
_____

Date:_____ **Daily Log** Overall Rating: 🙂 😐 ☹️

| Did you remember to take your medications today?

_____am/pm y/n
_____am/pm y/n
_____am/pm y/n
_____am/pm y/n
_____am/pm y/n | Off times: Time of day symptoms started: _____

Symptoms: Fatigue, Tremors, Mood Change, Sweating, Anxiety, Not Thinking Clearly, Feeling Restless (circle any that apply)
Other _____ |

Evaluate your sleep last night.
Scale : 0 1 2 3 4 5 (poor 0 to excellent 5)
Bad or disturbing dreams?_____

Dizziness? y/n _____
Falls? y/n _____
Depression? y/n _____   Alcohol? y/n
Hallucinations? y/n _____   How much?_____

Did you exercise today? y/n How Long? _____ minutes
Type of Exercise: _____

Did you eat three balanced healthy meals today?
Breakfast y/n _____
Lunch y/n _____
Dinner y/n _____

What did you accomplish today? _____
_____

Date:_____ **Daily Log** Overall Rating: 😊 😐 ☹️

| Did you remember to take your medications today?

_____am/pm y/n
_____am/pm y/n
_____am/pm y/n
_____am/pm y/n
_____am/pm y/n | Off times: Time of day symptoms started: _____

Symptoms: Fatigue, Tremors, Mood Change, Sweating, Anxiety, Not Thinking Clearly, Feeling Restless (circle any that apply)
Other _____ |

Evaluate your sleep last night.
Scale : 0 1 2 3 4 5 (poor 0 to excellent 5)
Bad or disturbing dreams?_____

Dizziness? y/n _____
Falls? y/n _____
Depression? y/n _____   Alcohol? y/n
Hallucinations? y/n _____   How much?_____

Did you exercise today? y/n How Long? _____ minutes
Type of Exercise: _____

Did you eat three balanced healthy meals today?
Breakfast y/n _____
Lunch y/n _____
Dinner y/n _____

What did you accomplish today? _____
_____

Date:_____ **Daily Log** Overall Rating: 🙂 😐 ☹

| Did you remember to take your medications today?

_____am/pm y/n
_____am/pm y/n
_____am/pm y/n
_____am/pm y/n
_____am/pm y/n | Off times: Time of day symptoms started: _____

Symptoms: Fatigue, Tremors, Mood Change, Sweating, Anxiety, Not Thinking Clearly, Feeling Restless (circle any that apply)
Other _____ |

Evaluate your sleep last night.
Scale : 0 1 2 3 4 5 (poor 0 to excellent 5)
Bad or disturbing dreams?_____

Dizziness? y/n _____
Falls? y/n _____
Depression? y/n _____   Alcohol? y/n
Hallucinations? y/n _____   How much?_____

Did you exercise today? y/n How Long? _____ minutes
Type of Exercise: _____

Did you eat three balanced healthy meals today?
Breakfast y/n _____
Lunch y/n _____
Dinner y/n _____

What did you accomplish today? _____
_____

Date:_____ **Daily Log**   Overall Rating: 😊 😐 ☹

| Did you remember to take your medications today?

_____am/pm y/n
_____am/pm y/n
_____am/pm y/n
_____am/pm y/n
_____am/pm y/n | Off times: Time of day symptoms started: _____

Symptoms: Fatigue, Tremors, Mood Change, Sweating, Anxiety, Not Thinking Clearly, Feeling Restless (circle any that apply)
Other _____ |

Evaluate your sleep last night.
Scale : 0 1 2 3 4 5   (poor 0 to excellent 5)
Bad or disturbing dreams?_____

Dizziness? y/n _____
Falls? y/n _____
Depression? y/n _____   Alcohol? y/n
Hallucinations? y/n _____   How much?_____

Did you exercise today? y/n How Long? _____ minutes
Type of Exercise: _____

Did you eat three balanced healthy meals today?
Breakfast y/n _____
Lunch y/n _____
Dinner y/n _____

What did you accomplish today? _____
_____

Date:_____   **Daily Log**   Overall Rating: 🙂 😐 ☹️

| Did you remember to take your medications today? _____am/pm y/n _____am/pm y/n _____am/pm y/n _____am/pm y/n _____am/pm y/n | Off times: Time of day symptoms started: _____ Symptoms: Fatigue, Tremors, Mood Change, Sweating, Anxiety, Not Thinking Clearly, Feeling Restless (circle any that apply) Other _____ |

Evaluate your sleep last night.
Scale : 0 1 2 3 4 5   (poor 0 to excellent 5)
Bad or disturbing dreams?_____

Dizziness? y/n _____
Falls? y/n _____
Depression? y/n _____   Alcohol? y/n
Hallucinations? y/n _____   How much?_____

Did you exercise today? y/n How Long? _____ minutes
Type of Exercise: _____

Did you eat three balanced healthy meals today?
Breakfast y/n _____
Lunch y/n _____
Dinner y/n _____

What did you accomplish today? _____
_____

Date:_____ **Daily Log** Overall Rating: ☺ 😐 ☹

Did you remember to take your medications today?

_____am/pm y/n
_____am/pm y/n
_____am/pm y/n
_____am/pm y/n
_____am/pm y/n

Off times: Time of day symptoms started: _____

Symptoms: Fatigue, Tremors, Mood Change, Sweating, Anxiety, Not Thinking Clearly, Feeling Restless (circle any that apply)
Other _____

Evaluate your sleep last night.
Scale : 0 1 2 3 4 5   (poor 0 to excellent 5)
Bad or disturbing dreams?_____

Dizziness? y/n _____
Falls? y/n _____
Depression? y/n _____   Alcohol? y/n
Hallucinations? y/n _____   How much?_____

Did you exercise today? y/n How Long? _____ minutes
Type of Exercise: _____

Did you eat three balanced healthy meals today?
Breakfast y/n _____
Lunch y/n _____
Dinner y/n _____

What did you accomplish today? _____
_____

Date:_____ **Daily Log**   Overall Rating: 😊 😐 ☹

Did you remember to take your medications today? _____am/pm y/n _____am/pm y/n _____am/pm y/n _____am/pm y/n _____am/pm y/n	Off times: Time of day symptoms started: _____ Symptoms: Fatigue, Tremors, Mood Change, Sweating, Anxiety, Not Thinking Clearly, Feeling Restless (circle any that apply) Other _____

Evaluate your sleep last night.
Scale : 0 1 2 3 4 5 (poor 0 to excellent 5)
Bad or disturbing dreams?_____

Dizziness? y/n _____
Falls? y/n _____
Depression? y/n _____   Alcohol? y/n
Hallucinations? y/n _____   How much?_____

Did you exercise today? y/n How Long? _____ minutes
Type of Exercise: _____

Did you eat three balanced healthy meals today?
Breakfast y/n _____
Lunch y/n _____
Dinner y/n _____

What did you accomplish today? _____
_____
_____

Date:_____ **Daily Log** Overall Rating: 😀 😐 ☹️

Did you remember to take your medications today?

_____ am/pm y/n
_____ am/pm y/n
_____ am/pm y/n
_____ am/pm y/n
_____ am/pm y/n

Off times: Time of day symptoms started: _____

Symptoms: Fatigue, Tremors, Mood Change, Sweating, Anxiety, Not Thinking Clearly, Feeling Restless (circle any that apply)
Other _____

Evaluate your sleep last night.
Scale : 0 1 2 3 4 5 (poor 0 to excellent 5)
Bad or disturbing dreams?_____

Dizziness? y/n _____
Falls? y/n _____
Depression? y/n _____
Hallucinations? y/n _____
Alcohol? y/n
How much?_____

Did you exercise today? y/n How Long? _____ minutes
Type of Exercise: _____

Did you eat three balanced healthy meals today?
Breakfast y/n _____
Lunch y/n _____
Dinner y/n _____

What did you accomplish today? _____
_____

Date:_____   **Daily Log**   Overall Rating: 🙂 😐 ☹️

Did you remember to take your medications today?

_____am/pm y/n
_____am/pm y/n
_____am/pm y/n
_____am/pm y/n
_____am/pm y/n

Off times: Time of day symptoms started: _____

Symptoms: Fatigue, Tremors, Mood Change, Sweating, Anxiety, Not Thinking Clearly, Feeling Restless (circle any that apply)
Other _____

Evaluate your sleep last night.
Scale : 0 1 2 3 4 5 (poor 0 to excellent 5)
Bad or disturbing dreams?_____

Dizziness? y/n _____
Falls? y/n _____
Depression? y/n _____   Alcohol? y/n
Hallucinations? y/n _____   How much?_____

Did you exercise today? y/n How Long? _____ minutes
Type of Exercise: _____

Did you eat three balanced healthy meals today?
Breakfast y/n _____
Lunch y/n _____
Dinner y/n _____

What did you accomplish today? _____
_____

Date:_____ **Daily Log**   Overall Rating: ☺ 😐 ☹

| Did you remember to take your medications today?

_____am/pm y/n
_____am/pm y/n
_____am/pm y/n
_____am/pm y/n
_____am/pm y/n | Off times: Time of day symptoms started: _____

Symptoms: Fatigue, Tremors, Mood Change, Sweating, Anxiety, Not Thinking Clearly, Feeling Restless (circle any that apply)
Other _____ |

Evaluate your sleep last night.
Scale : 0 1 2 3 4 5 (poor 0 to excellent 5)
Bad or disturbing dreams?_____

Dizziness? y/n _____
Falls? y/n _____
Depression? y/n _____   Alcohol? y/n
Hallucinations? y/n _____   How much?_____

Did you exercise today? y/n How Long? _____ minutes
Type of Exercise: _____

Did you eat three balanced healthy meals today?
Breakfast y/n _____
Lunch y/n _____
Dinner y/n _____

What did you accomplish today? _____
_____

Date:_____   **Daily Log**   Overall Rating: 😊 😐 ☹

| Did you remember to take your medications today?

_____am/pm y/n
_____am/pm y/n
_____am/pm y/n
_____am/pm y/n
_____am/pm y/n | Off times: Time of day symptoms started: _____

Symptoms: Fatigue, Tremors, Mood Change, Sweating, Anxiety, Not Thinking Clearly, Feeling Restless (circle any that apply)
Other _____ |

Evaluate your sleep last night.
Scale : 0 1 2 3 4 5 (poor 0 to excellent 5)
Bad or disturbing dreams?_____

Dizziness? y/n _____
Falls? y/n _____
Depression? y/n _____   Alcohol? y/n
Hallucinations? y/n _____   How much?_____

Did you exercise today? y/n How Long? _____ minutes
Type of Exercise: _____

Did you eat three balanced healthy meals today?
Breakfast y/n _____
Lunch y/n _____
Dinner y/n _____

What did you accomplish today? _____
_____

Date:_____   **Daily Log**   Overall Rating: 😊 😐 ☹️

Did you remember to take your medications today?

_____am/pm y/n
_____am/pm y/n
_____am/pm y/n
_____am/pm y/n
_____am/pm y/n

Off times: Time of day symptoms started: _____

Symptoms: Fatigue, Tremors, Mood Change, Sweating, Anxiety, Not Thinking Clearly, Feeling Restless (circle any that apply)
Other _____

Evaluate your sleep last night.
Scale : 0 1 2 3 4 5 (poor 0 to excellent 5)
Bad or disturbing dreams?_____

Dizziness? y/n _____
Falls? y/n _____
Depression? y/n _____   Alcohol? y/n
Hallucinations? y/n _____   How much?_____

Did you exercise today? y/n How Long? _____ minutes
Type of Exercise: _____

Did you eat three balanced healthy meals today?
Breakfast y/n _____
Lunch y/n _____
Dinner y/n _____

What did you accomplish today? _____
_____

Date:_____ **Daily Log** Overall Rating: 😊 😐 ☹️

Did you remember to take your medications today?	Off times: Time of day symptoms started: _____
_____am/pm y/n _____am/pm y/n _____am/pm y/n _____am/pm y/n _____am/pm y/n	Symptoms: Fatigue, Tremors, Mood Change, Sweating, Anxiety, Not Thinking Clearly, Feeling Restless (circle any that apply) Other _____

Evaluate your sleep last night.
Scale : 0 1 2 3 4 5 (poor 0 to excellent 5)
Bad or disturbing dreams?_____

Dizziness? y/n _____
Falls? y/n _____
Depression? y/n _____   Alcohol? y/n
Hallucinations? y/n _____   How much?_____

Did you exercise today? y/n How Long? _____ minutes
Type of Exercise: _____

Did you eat three balanced healthy meals today?
Breakfast y/n _____
Lunch y/n _____
Dinner y/n _____

What did you accomplish today? _____
_____

Date:_____   **Daily Log**   Overall Rating: 😊 😐 ☹️

| Did you remember to take your medications today?

_____am/pm y/n
_____am/pm y/n
_____am/pm y/n
_____am/pm y/n
_____am/pm y/n | Off times: Time of day symptoms started: _____

Symptoms: Fatigue, Tremors, Mood Change, Sweating, Anxiety, Not Thinking Clearly, Feeling Restless (circle any that apply)
Other _____ |

Evaluate your sleep last night.
Scale : 0 1 2 3 4 5   (poor 0 to excellent 5)
Bad or disturbing dreams?_____

Dizziness? y/n _____
Falls? y/n _____
Depression? y/n _____   Alcohol? y/n
Hallucinations? y/n _____   How much?_____

Did you exercise today? y/n How Long? _____ minutes
Type of Exercise: _____

Did you eat three balanced healthy meals today?
Breakfast y/n _____
Lunch y/n _____
Dinner y/n _____

What did you accomplish today? _____
_____

Date:_____   **Daily Log**   Overall Rating: 😊 😐 ☹

Did you remember to take your medications today?	Off times: Time of day symptoms started: _____
_____am/pm y/n _____am/pm y/n _____am/pm y/n _____am/pm y/n _____am/pm y/n	Symptoms: Fatigue, Tremors, Mood Change, Sweating, Anxiety, Not Thinking Clearly, Feeling Restless (circle any that apply) Other _____

Evaluate your sleep last night.
Scale : 0 1 2 3 4 5 (poor 0 to excellent 5)
Bad or disturbing dreams?_____

Dizziness? y/n _____
Falls? y/n _____
Depression? y/n _____   Alcohol? y/n
Hallucinations? y/n _____   How much?_____

Did you exercise today? y/n How Long? _____ minutes
Type of Exercise: _____

Did you eat three balanced healthy meals today?
Breakfast y/n _____
Lunch y/n _____
Dinner y/n _____

What did you accomplish today? _____
_____

Date:_____ **Daily Log** Overall Rating: 😊 😐 ☹

| Did you remember to take your medications today?

_____am/pm y/n
_____am/pm y/n
_____am/pm y/n
_____am/pm y/n
_____am/pm y/n | Off times: Time of day symptoms started: _____

Symptoms: Fatigue, Tremors, Mood Change, Sweating, Anxiety, Not Thinking Clearly, Feeling Restless (circle any that apply)
Other _____ |

Evaluate your sleep last night.
Scale : 0 1 2 3 4 5 (poor 0 to excellent 5)
Bad or disturbing dreams?_____

Dizziness? y/n _____
Falls? y/n _____
Depression? y/n _____   Alcohol? y/n
Hallucinations? y/n _____   How much?_____

Did you exercise today? y/n How Long? _____ minutes
Type of Exercise: _____

Did you eat three balanced healthy meals today?
Breakfast y/n _____
Lunch y/n _____
Dinner y/n _____

What did you accomplish today? _____
_____

Date:_____ **Daily Log** Overall Rating: 🙂 😐 ☹️

Did you remember to take your medications today?	Off times: Time of day symptoms started: _____
_____am/pm y/n _____am/pm y/n _____am/pm y/n _____am/pm y/n _____am/pm y/n	Symptoms: Fatigue, Tremors, Mood Change, Sweating, Anxiety, Not Thinking Clearly, Feeling Restless (circle any that apply) Other _____

Evaluate your sleep last night.
Scale : 0 1 2 3 4 5 (poor 0 to excellent 5)
Bad or disturbing dreams?_____

Dizziness? y/n _____
Falls? y/n _____
Depression? y/n _____   Alcohol? y/n
Hallucinations? y/n _____   How much?_____

Did you exercise today? y/n How Long? _____ minutes
Type of Exercise: _____

Did you eat three balanced healthy meals today?
Breakfast y/n _____
Lunch y/n _____
Dinner y/n _____

What did you accomplish today? _____
_____

Date:_____   **Daily Log**   Overall Rating: 😊 😐 ☹

| Did you remember to take your medications today?

_____am/pm y/n
_____am/pm y/n
_____am/pm y/n
_____am/pm y/n
_____am/pm y/n | Off times: Time of day symptoms started: _____

Symptoms: Fatigue, Tremors, Mood Change, Sweating, Anxiety, Not Thinking Clearly, Feeling Restless (circle any that apply)
Other _____ |

Evaluate your sleep last night.
Scale : 0 1 2 3 4 5 (poor 0 to excellent 5)
Bad or disturbing dreams?_____

Dizziness? y/n _____
Falls? y/n _____
Depression? y/n _____   Alcohol? y/n
Hallucinations? y/n _____   How much?_____

Did you exercise today? y/n How Long? _____ minutes
Type of Exercise: _____

Did you eat three balanced healthy meals today?
Breakfast y/n _____
Lunch y/n _____
Dinner y/n _____

What did you accomplish today? _____
_____

Date:_____ **Daily Log** Overall Rating: 😊 😐 ☹️

| Did you remember to take your medications today?

_____am/pm y/n
_____am/pm y/n
_____am/pm y/n
_____am/pm y/n
_____am/pm y/n | Off times: Time of day symptoms started: _____

Symptoms: Fatigue, Tremors, Mood Change, Sweating, Anxiety, Not Thinking Clearly, Feeling Restless (circle any that apply)
Other _____ |

Evaluate your sleep last night.
Scale : 0 1 2 3 4 5 (poor 0 to excellent 5)
Bad or disturbing dreams?_____

Dizziness? y/n _____
Falls? y/n _____
Depression? y/n _____   Alcohol? y/n
Hallucinations? y/n _____   How much?_____

Did you exercise today? y/n How Long? _____ minutes
Type of Exercise: _____

Did you eat three balanced healthy meals today?
Breakfast y/n _____
Lunch y/n _____
Dinner y/n _____

What did you accomplish today? _____
_____

Date:_____ **Daily Log** Overall Rating: 😊 😐 ☹

| Did you remember to take your medications today?

_____am/pm y/n
_____am/pm y/n
_____am/pm y/n
_____am/pm y/n
_____am/pm y/n | Off times: Time of day symptoms started: _____

Symptoms: Fatigue, Tremors, Mood Change, Sweating, Anxiety, Not Thinking Clearly, Feeling Restless (circle any that apply)
Other _____ |

Evaluate your sleep last night.
Scale : 0 1 2 3 4 5 (poor 0 to excellent 5)
Bad or disturbing dreams?_____

Dizziness? y/n _____
Falls? y/n _____
Depression? y/n _____   Alcohol? y/n
Hallucinations? y/n _____   How much?_____

Did you exercise today? y/n How Long? _____ minutes
Type of Exercise: _____

Did you eat three balanced healthy meals today?
Breakfast y/n _____
Lunch y/n _____
Dinner y/n _____

What did you accomplish today? _____
_____

Date:_____ **Daily Log** Overall Rating: 😊 😐 ☹

| Did you remember to take your medications today?

_____am/pm y/n
_____am/pm y/n
_____am/pm y/n
_____am/pm y/n
_____am/pm y/n | Off times: Time of day symptoms started: _____

Symptoms: Fatigue, Tremors, Mood Change, Sweating, Anxiety, Not Thinking Clearly, Feeling Restless (circle any that apply)
Other _____ |

Evaluate your sleep last night.
Scale : 0 1 2 3 4 5 (poor 0 to excellent 5)
Bad or disturbing dreams?_____

Dizziness? y/n _____
Falls? y/n _____
Depression? y/n _____   Alcohol? y/n
Hallucinations? y/n _____   How much?_____

Did you exercise today? y/n How Long? _____ minutes
Type of Exercise: _____

Did you eat three balanced healthy meals today?
Breakfast y/n _____
Lunch y/n _____
Dinner y/n _____

What did you accomplish today? _____
_____

Date:_____ **Daily Log** Overall Rating: 😊 😐 ☹️

| Did you remember to take your medications today? _____am/pm y/n _____am/pm y/n _____am/pm y/n _____am/pm y/n _____am/pm y/n | Off times: Time of day symptoms started: _____ Symptoms: Fatigue, Tremors, Mood Change, Sweating, Anxiety, Not Thinking Clearly, Feeling Restless (circle any that apply) Other _____ |

Evaluate your sleep last night.
Scale : 0 1 2 3 4 5 (poor 0 to excellent 5)
Bad or disturbing dreams?_____

Dizziness? y/n _____
Falls? y/n _____
Depression? y/n _____   Alcohol? y/n
Hallucinations? y/n _____   How much?_____

Did you exercise today? y/n How Long? _____ minutes
Type of Exercise: _____

Did you eat three balanced healthy meals today?
Breakfast y/n _____
Lunch y/n _____
Dinner y/n _____

What did you accomplish today? _____
_____

Date:_____   **Daily Log**   Overall Rating: 😊 😐 ☹

Did you remember to take your medications today?

_____am/pm y/n
_____am/pm y/n
_____am/pm y/n
_____am/pm y/n
_____am/pm y/n

Off times: Time of day symptoms started: _____

Symptoms: Fatigue, Tremors, Mood Change, Sweating, Anxiety, Not Thinking Clearly, Feeling Restless (circle any that apply)
Other _____

Evaluate your sleep last night.
Scale : 0 1 2 3 4 5 (poor 0 to excellent 5)
Bad or disturbing dreams?_____

Dizziness? y/n _____
Falls? y/n _____
Depression? y/n _____   Alcohol? y/n
Hallucinations? y/n _____   How much?_____

Did you exercise today? y/n How Long? _____ minutes
Type of Exercise: _____

Did you eat three balanced healthy meals today?
Breakfast y/n _____
Lunch y/n _____
Dinner y/n _____

What did you accomplish today? _____
_____

Date:_____ **Daily Log** Overall Rating: 😊 😐 ☹

| Did you remember to take your medications today?

_____am/pm y/n
_____am/pm y/n
_____am/pm y/n
_____am/pm y/n
_____am/pm y/n | Off times: Time of day symptoms started: _____

Symptoms: Fatigue, Tremors, Mood Change, Sweating, Anxiety, Not Thinking Clearly, Feeling Restless (circle any that apply)
Other _____ |

Evaluate your sleep last night.
Scale : 0 1 2 3 4 5 (poor 0 to excellent 5)
Bad or disturbing dreams?_____

Dizziness? y/n _____
Falls? y/n _____
Depression? y/n _____ Alcohol? y/n
Hallucinations? y/n _____ How much?_____

Did you exercise today? y/n How Long? _____ minutes
Type of Exercise: _____

Did you eat three balanced healthy meals today?
Breakfast y/n _____
Lunch y/n _____
Dinner y/n _____

What did you accomplish today? _____
_____

Date:_____ **Daily Log** Overall Rating: 🙂 😐 ☹️

| Did you remember to take your medications today?

_____am/pm y/n
_____am/pm y/n
_____am/pm y/n
_____am/pm y/n
_____am/pm y/n | Off times: Time of day symptoms started: _____

Symptoms: Fatigue, Tremors, Mood Change, Sweating, Anxiety, Not Thinking Clearly, Feeling Restless (circle any that apply)
Other _____ |

Evaluate your sleep last night.
Scale : 0 1 2 3 4 5 (poor 0 to excellent 5)
Bad or disturbing dreams?_____

Dizziness? y/n _____
Falls? y/n _____
Depression? y/n _____   Alcohol? y/n
Hallucinations? y/n _____   How much?_____

Did you exercise today? y/n How Long? _____ minutes
Type of Exercise: _____

Did you eat three balanced healthy meals today?
Breakfast y/n _____
Lunch y/n _____
Dinner y/n _____

What did you accomplish today? _____
_____

Date:_____ **Daily Log** Overall Rating: 😊 😐 ☹️

| Did you remember to take your medications today?

_____am/pm y/n
_____am/pm y/n
_____am/pm y/n
_____am/pm y/n
_____am/pm y/n | Off times: Time of day symptoms started: _____

Symptoms: Fatigue, Tremors, Mood Change, Sweating, Anxiety, Not Thinking Clearly, Feeling Restless (circle any that apply)
Other _____ |

Evaluate your sleep last night.
Scale : 0 1 2 3 4 5 (poor 0 to excellent 5)
Bad or disturbing dreams?_____

Dizziness? y/n _____
Falls? y/n _____
Depression? y/n _____   Alcohol? y/n
Hallucinations? y/n _____   How much?_____

Did you exercise today? y/n How Long? _____ minutes
Type of Exercise: _____

Did you eat three balanced healthy meals today?
Breakfast y/n _____
Lunch y/n _____
Dinner y/n _____

What did you accomplish today? _____
_____

Date:_____ **Daily Log** Overall Rating: 😊 😐 ☹

Did you remember to take your medications today?

_____am/pm y/n
_____am/pm y/n
_____am/pm y/n
_____am/pm y/n
_____am/pm y/n

Off times: Time of day symptoms started: _____

Symptoms: Fatigue, Tremors, Mood Change, Sweating, Anxiety, Not Thinking Clearly, Feeling Restless (circle any that apply)
Other _____

Evaluate your sleep last night.
Scale : 0 1 2 3 4 5 (poor 0 to excellent 5)
Bad or disturbing dreams?_____

Dizziness? y/n _____
Falls? y/n _____
Depression? y/n _____
Hallucinations? y/n _____

Alcohol? y/n
How much?_____

Did you exercise today? y/n How Long? _____ minutes
Type of Exercise: _____

Did you eat three balanced healthy meals today?
Breakfast y/n _____
Lunch y/n _____
Dinner y/n _____

What did you accomplish today? _____
_____

Date:_____ **Daily Log** Overall Rating: ☺ 😐 ☹

| Did you remember to take your medications today?

_____am/pm y/n
_____am/pm y/n
_____am/pm y/n
_____am/pm y/n
_____am/pm y/n | Off times: Time of day symptoms started: _____

Symptoms: Fatigue, Tremors, Mood Change, Sweating, Anxiety, Not Thinking Clearly, Feeling Restless (circle any that apply)
Other _____ |

Evaluate your sleep last night.
Scale : 0 1 2 3 4 5 (poor 0 to excellent 5)
Bad or disturbing dreams?_____

Dizziness? y/n _____
Falls? y/n _____
Depression? y/n _____   Alcohol? y/n
Hallucinations? y/n _____   How much?_____

Did you exercise today? y/n How Long? _____ minutes
Type of Exercise: _____

Did you eat three balanced healthy meals today?
Breakfast y/n _____
Lunch y/n _____
Dinner y/n _____

What did you accomplish today? _____
_____

Date:_____   **Daily Log**   Overall Rating: ☺ 😐 ☹

Did you remember to take your medications today?	Off times: Time of day symptoms started: _____
_____am/pm y/n _____am/pm y/n _____am/pm y/n _____am/pm y/n _____am/pm y/n	Symptoms: Fatigue, Tremors, Mood Change, Sweating, Anxiety, Not Thinking Clearly, Feeling Restless (circle any that apply) Other _____

Evaluate your sleep last night.
Scale : 0 1 2 3 4 5 (poor 0 to excellent 5)
Bad or disturbing dreams?_____

Dizziness? y/n _____
Falls? y/n _____
Depression? y/n _____   Alcohol? y/n
Hallucinations? y/n _____   How much?_____

Did you exercise today? y/n How Long? _____ minutes
Type of Exercise: _____

Did you eat three balanced healthy meals today?
Breakfast y/n _____
Lunch y/n _____
Dinner y/n _____

What did you accomplish today? _____
_____

Date:_____ **Daily Log** Overall Rating: 😊 😐 ☹

Did you remember to take your medications today?

_____ am/pm y/n
_____ am/pm y/n
_____ am/pm y/n
_____ am/pm y/n
_____ am/pm y/n

Off times: Time of day symptoms started: _____

Symptoms: Fatigue, Tremors, Mood Change, Sweating, Anxiety, Not Thinking Clearly, Feeling Restless (circle any that apply)
Other _____

Evaluate your sleep last night.
Scale : 0 1 2 3 4 5   (poor 0 to excellent 5)
Bad or disturbing dreams?_____

Dizziness? y/n _____
Falls? y/n _____
Depression? y/n _____   Alcohol? y/n
Hallucinations? y/n _____   How much?_____

Did you exercise today? y/n How Long? _____ minutes
Type of Exercise: _____

Did you eat three balanced healthy meals today?
Breakfast y/n _____
Lunch y/n _____
Dinner y/n _____

What did you accomplish today? _____
_____

Date:_____ **Daily Log** Overall Rating: 😊 😐 ☹

| Did you remember to take your medications today?

_____am/pm y/n
_____am/pm y/n
_____am/pm y/n
_____am/pm y/n
_____am/pm y/n | Off times: Time of day symptoms started: _____

Symptoms: Fatigue, Tremors, Mood Change, Sweating, Anxiety, Not Thinking Clearly, Feeling Restless (circle any that apply)
Other _____ |

Evaluate your sleep last night.
Scale : 0 1 2 3 4 5   (poor 0 to excellent 5)
Bad or disturbing dreams?_____

Dizziness? y/n _____
Falls? y/n _____
Depression? y/n _____   Alcohol? y/n
Hallucinations? y/n _____   How much?_____

Did you exercise today? y/n How Long? _____ minutes
Type of Exercise: _____

Did you eat three balanced healthy meals today?
Breakfast y/n _____
Lunch y/n _____
Dinner y/n _____

What did you accomplish today? _____
_____

Date:_____   **Daily Log**   Overall Rating: 😊 😐 ☹

| Did you remember to take your medications today?

_____am/pm y/n
_____am/pm y/n
_____am/pm y/n
_____am/pm y/n
_____am/pm y/n | Off times: Time of day symptoms started: _____

Symptoms: Fatigue, Tremors, Mood Change, Sweating, Anxiety, Not Thinking Clearly, Feeling Restless (circle any that apply)
Other _____ |

Evaluate your sleep last night.
Scale : 0 1 2 3 4 5 (poor 0 to excellent 5)
Bad or disturbing dreams?_____

Dizziness? y/n _____
Falls? y/n _____
Depression? y/n _____   Alcohol? y/n
Hallucinations? y/n _____   How much?_____

Did you exercise today? y/n How Long? _____ minutes
Type of Exercise: _____

Did you eat three balanced healthy meals today?
Breakfast y/n _____
Lunch y/n _____
Dinner y/n _____

What did you accomplish today? _____
_____

Date:_____ **Daily Log** Overall Rating: 😊 😐 ☹

Did you remember to take your medications today? _____am/pm y/n _____am/pm y/n _____am/pm y/n _____am/pm y/n _____am/pm y/n	Off times: Time of day symptoms started: _____ Symptoms: Fatigue, Tremors, Mood Change, Sweating, Anxiety, Not Thinking Clearly, Feeling Restless (circle any that apply) Other _____

Evaluate your sleep last night.
Scale : 0 1 2 3 4 5 (poor 0 to excellent 5)
Bad or disturbing dreams?_____

Dizziness? y/n _____
Falls? y/n _____
Depression? y/n _____   Alcohol? y/n
Hallucinations? y/n _____   How much?_____

Did you exercise today? y/n How Long? _____ minutes
Type of Exercise: _____

Did you eat three balanced healthy meals today?
Breakfast y/n _____
Lunch y/n _____
Dinner y/n _____

What did you accomplish today? _____
_____

Date:_____ **Daily Log** Overall Rating: 😊 😐 ☹

Did you remember to take your medications today?

_____am/pm y/n
_____am/pm y/n
_____am/pm y/n
_____am/pm y/n
_____am/pm y/n

Off times: Time of day symptoms started: _____

Symptoms: Fatigue, Tremors, Mood Change, Sweating, Anxiety, Not Thinking Clearly, Feeling Restless (circle any that apply)
Other _____

Evaluate your sleep last night.
Scale: 0 1 2 3 4 5 (poor 0 to excellent 5)
Bad or disturbing dreams?_____

Dizziness? y/n _____
Falls? y/n _____
Depression? y/n _____   Alcohol? y/n
Hallucinations? y/n _____ How much?_____

Did you exercise today? y/n How Long? _____ minutes
Type of Exercise: _____

Did you eat three balanced healthy meals today?
Breakfast y/n _____
Lunch y/n _____
Dinner y/n _____

What did you accomplish today? _____
_____

Date:_____   **Daily Log**   Overall Rating: ☺ 😐 ☹

| Did you remember to take your medications today?

_____am/pm y/n
_____am/pm y/n
_____am/pm y/n
_____am/pm y/n
_____am/pm y/n | Off times: Time of day symptoms started: _____

Symptoms: Fatigue, Tremors, Mood Change, Sweating, Anxiety, Not Thinking Clearly, Feeling Restless (circle any that apply)
Other _____ |

Evaluate your sleep last night.
Scale : 0 1 2 3 4 5 (poor 0 to excellent 5)
Bad or disturbing dreams?_____

Dizziness? y/n _____
Falls? y/n _____
Depression? y/n _____   Alcohol? y/n
Hallucinations? y/n _____   How much?_____

Did you exercise today? y/n How Long? _____ minutes
Type of Exercise: _____

Did you eat three balanced healthy meals today?
Breakfast y/n _____
Lunch y/n _____
Dinner y/n _____

What did you accomplish today? _____
_____

Date:_____ **Daily Log** Overall Rating: 😊 😐 ☹

Did you remember to take your medications today?	Off times: Time of day symptoms started: _____
_____am/pm y/n _____am/pm y/n _____am/pm y/n _____am/pm y/n _____am/pm y/n	Symptoms: Fatigue, Tremors, Mood Change, Sweating, Anxiety, Not Thinking Clearly, Feeling Restless (circle any that apply) Other _____

Evaluate your sleep last night.
Scale : 0 1 2 3 4 5 (poor 0 to excellent 5)
Bad or disturbing dreams?_____

Dizziness? y/n _____
Falls? y/n _____
Depression? y/n _____   Alcohol? y/n
Hallucinations? y/n _____   How much?_____

Did you exercise today? y/n How Long? _____ minutes
Type of Exercise: _____

Did you eat three balanced healthy meals today?
Breakfast y/n _____
Lunch y/n _____
Dinner y/n _____

What did you accomplish today? _____
_____

Date:_____ **Daily Log** Overall Rating: 😊 😐 ☹️

| Did you remember to take your medications today?

_____am/pm y/n
_____am/pm y/n
_____am/pm y/n
_____am/pm y/n
_____am/pm y/n | Off times: Time of day symptoms started: _____

Symptoms: Fatigue, Tremors, Mood Change, Sweating, Anxiety, Not Thinking Clearly, Feeling Restless (circle any that apply)
Other _____ |

Evaluate your sleep last night.
Scale : 0 1 2 3 4 5 (poor 0 to excellent 5)
Bad or disturbing dreams?_____

Dizziness? y/n _____
Falls? y/n _____
Depression? y/n _____   Alcohol? y/n
Hallucinations? y/n _____   How much?_____

Did you exercise today? y/n How Long? _____ minutes
Type of Exercise: _____

Did you eat three balanced healthy meals today?
Breakfast y/n _____
Lunch y/n _____
Dinner y/n _____

What did you accomplish today? _____
_____

Date:_____ **Daily Log**   Overall Rating: 😊 😐 ☹

| Did you remember to take your medications today?

 _____am/pm y/n
 _____am/pm y/n
 _____am/pm y/n
 _____am/pm y/n
 _____am/pm y/n | Off times: Time of day symptoms started: _____

 Symptoms: Fatigue, Tremors, Mood Change, Sweating, Anxiety, Not Thinking Clearly, Feeling Restless (circle any that apply)
 Other _____ |

Evaluate your sleep last night.
Scale : 0 1 2 3 4 5 (poor 0 to excellent 5)
Bad or disturbing dreams?_____

Dizziness? y/n _____
Falls? y/n _____
Depression? y/n _____   Alcohol? y/n
Hallucinations? y/n _____   How much?_____

Did you exercise today? y/n How Long? _____ minutes
Type of Exercise: _____

Did you eat three balanced healthy meals today?
Breakfast y/n _____
Lunch y/n _____
Dinner y/n _____

What did you accomplish today? _____
_____

Date:_____ **Daily Log** Overall Rating: 🙂 😐 ☹️

Did you remember to take your medications today?	Off times: Time of day symptoms started: _____
_____am/pm y/n _____am/pm y/n _____am/pm y/n _____am/pm y/n _____am/pm y/n	Symptoms: Fatigue, Tremors, Mood Change, Sweating, Anxiety, Not Thinking Clearly, Feeling Restless (circle any that apply) Other _____

Evaluate your sleep last night.
Scale : 0 1 2 3 4 5 (poor 0 to excellent 5)
Bad or disturbing dreams?_____

Dizziness? y/n _____
Falls? y/n _____
Depression? y/n _____   Alcohol? y/n
Hallucinations? y/n _____   How much?_____

Did you exercise today? y/n How Long? _____ minutes
Type of Exercise: _____

Did you eat three balanced healthy meals today?
Breakfast y/n _____
Lunch y/n _____
Dinner y/n _____

What did you accomplish today? _____
_____

Date:_____ **Daily Log** Overall Rating: 🙂 😐 ☹️

| Did you remember to take your medications today?

 _____am/pm y/n
 _____am/pm y/n
 _____am/pm y/n
 _____am/pm y/n
 _____am/pm y/n | Off times: Time of day symptoms started: _____

 Symptoms: Fatigue, Tremors, Mood Change, Sweating, Anxiety, Not Thinking Clearly, Feeling Restless (circle any that apply)
 Other _____ |

Evaluate your sleep last night.
Scale : 0 1 2 3 4 5 (poor 0 to excellent 5)
Bad or disturbing dreams?_____

Dizziness? y/n _____
Falls? y/n _____
Depression? y/n _____   Alcohol? y/n
Hallucinations? y/n _____   How much?_____

Did you exercise today? y/n How Long? _____ minutes
Type of Exercise: _____

Did you eat three balanced healthy meals today?
Breakfast y/n _____
Lunch y/n _____
Dinner y/n _____

What did you accomplish today? _____
_____

Date:_____ **Daily Log** Overall Rating: 😊 😐 ☹️

Did you remember to take your medications today?

_____am/pm y/n
_____am/pm y/n
_____am/pm y/n
_____am/pm y/n
_____am/pm y/n

Off times: Time of day symptoms started: _____

Symptoms: Fatigue, Tremors, Mood Change, Sweating, Anxiety, Not Thinking Clearly, Feeling Restless (circle any that apply)
Other _____

Evaluate your sleep last night.
Scale : 0 1 2 3 4 5 (poor 0 to excellent 5)
Bad or disturbing dreams?_____

Dizziness? y/n _____
Falls? y/n _____
Depression? y/n _____   Alcohol? y/n
Hallucinations? y/n _____   How much?_____

Did you exercise today? y/n How Long? _____ minutes
Type of Exercise: _____

Did you eat three balanced healthy meals today?
Breakfast y/n _____
Lunch y/n _____
Dinner y/n _____

What did you accomplish today? _____
_____

Date:_____ **Daily Log** Overall Rating: 😊 😐 ☹

| Did you remember to take your medications today?

_____am/pm y/n
_____am/pm y/n
_____am/pm y/n
_____am/pm y/n
_____am/pm y/n | Off times: Time of day symptoms started: _____

Symptoms: Fatigue, Tremors, Mood Change, Sweating, Anxiety, Not Thinking Clearly, Feeling Restless (circle any that apply)
Other _____ |

Evaluate your sleep last night.
Scale : 0 1 2 3 4 5   (poor 0 to excellent 5)
Bad or disturbing dreams?_____

Dizziness? y/n _____
Falls? y/n _____
Depression? y/n _____   Alcohol? y/n
Hallucinations? y/n _____   How much?_____

Did you exercise today? y/n How Long? _____ minutes
Type of Exercise: _____

Did you eat three balanced healthy meals today?
Breakfast y/n _____
Lunch y/n _____
Dinner y/n _____

What did you accomplish today? _____
_____

Date:_____ **Daily Log** Overall Rating: 😊 😐 ☹

| Did you remember to take your medications today? _____am/pm y/n _____am/pm y/n _____am/pm y/n _____am/pm y/n _____am/pm y/n | Off times: Time of day symptoms started: _____ Symptoms: Fatigue, Tremors, Mood Change, Sweating, Anxiety, Not Thinking Clearly, Feeling Restless (circle any that apply) Other _____ |

Evaluate your sleep last night.
Scale : 0 1 2 3 4 5 (poor 0 to excellent 5)
Bad or disturbing dreams?_____

Dizziness? y/n _____
Falls? y/n _____
Depression? y/n _____   Alcohol? y/n
Hallucinations? y/n _____   How much?_____

Did you exercise today? y/n How Long? _____ minutes
Type of Exercise: _____

Did you eat three balanced healthy meals today?
Breakfast y/n _____
Lunch y/n _____
Dinner y/n _____

What did you accomplish today? _____
_____

Date:_____   **Daily Log**   Overall Rating: ☺ 😐 ☹

| Did you remember to take your medications today?

_____am/pm y/n
_____am/pm y/n
_____am/pm y/n
_____am/pm y/n
_____am/pm y/n | Off times: Time of day symptoms started: _____

Symptoms: Fatigue, Tremors, Mood Change, Sweating, Anxiety, Not Thinking Clearly, Feeling Restless (circle any that apply)
Other _____ |

Evaluate your sleep last night.
Scale : 0 1 2 3 4 5   (poor 0 to excellent 5)
Bad or disturbing dreams?_____

Dizziness? y/n _____
Falls? y/n _____
Depression? y/n _____   Alcohol? y/n
Hallucinations? y/n _____   How much?_____

Did you exercise today? y/n How Long? _____ minutes
Type of Exercise: _____

Did you eat three balanced healthy meals today?
Breakfast y/n _____
Lunch y/n _____
Dinner y/n _____

What did you accomplish today? _____
_____

Date:_____ **Daily Log** Overall Rating: 😊 😐 ☹️

| Did you remember to take your medications today?

_____am/pm y/n
_____am/pm y/n
_____am/pm y/n
_____am/pm y/n
_____am/pm y/n | Off times: Time of day symptoms started: _____

Symptoms: Fatigue, Tremors, Mood Change, Sweating, Anxiety, Not Thinking Clearly, Feeling Restless (circle any that apply)
Other _____ |

Evaluate your sleep last night.
Scale : 0 1 2 3 4 5 (poor 0 to excellent 5)
Bad or disturbing dreams?_____

Dizziness? y/n _____
Falls? y/n _____
Depression? y/n _____   Alcohol? y/n
Hallucinations? y/n _____   How much?_____

Did you exercise today? y/n How Long? _____ minutes
Type of Exercise: _____

Did you eat three balanced healthy meals today?
Breakfast y/n _____
Lunch y/n _____
Dinner y/n _____

What did you accomplish today? _____
_____

Date:_____ **Daily Log** Overall Rating: 😊 😐 ☹

| Did you remember to take your medications today?

_____am/pm y/n
_____am/pm y/n
_____am/pm y/n
_____am/pm y/n
_____am/pm y/n | Off times: Time of day symptoms started: _____

Symptoms: Fatigue, Tremors, Mood Change, Sweating, Anxiety, Not Thinking Clearly, Feeling Restless (circle any that apply)
Other _____ |

Evaluate your sleep last night.
Scale : 0 1 2 3 4 5 (poor 0 to excellent 5)
Bad or disturbing dreams?_____

Dizziness? y/n _____
Falls? y/n _____
Depression? y/n _____   Alcohol? y/n
Hallucinations? y/n _____   How much?_____

Did you exercise today? y/n How Long? _____ minutes
Type of Exercise: _____

Did you eat three balanced healthy meals today?
Breakfast y/n _____
Lunch y/n _____
Dinner y/n _____

What did you accomplish today? _____
_____

Date:_____ **Daily Log** Overall Rating: 😊 😐 ☹

| Did you remember to take your medications today?

_____ am/pm y/n
_____ am/pm y/n
_____ am/pm y/n
_____ am/pm y/n
_____ am/pm y/n | Off times: Time of day symptoms started: _____

Symptoms: Fatigue, Tremors, Mood Change, Sweating, Anxiety, Not Thinking Clearly, Feeling Restless (circle any that apply)
Other _____ |

Evaluate your sleep last night.
Scale : 0 1 2 3 4 5   (poor 0 to excellent 5)
Bad or disturbing dreams?_____

Dizziness? y/n _____
Falls? y/n _____
Depression? y/n _____   Alcohol? y/n
Hallucinations? y/n _____ How much?_____

Did you exercise today? y/n How Long? _____ minutes
Type of Exercise: _____

Did you eat three balanced healthy meals today?
Breakfast y/n _____
Lunch y/n _____
Dinner y/n _____

What did you accomplish today? _____
_____

Date:_____ **Daily Log** Overall Rating: 😊 😐 ☹

| Did you remember to take your medications today?

_____am/pm y/n
_____am/pm y/n
_____am/pm y/n
_____am/pm y/n
_____am/pm y/n | Off times: Time of day symptoms started: _____

Symptoms: Fatigue, Tremors, Mood Change, Sweating, Anxiety, Not Thinking Clearly, Feeling Restless (circle any that apply)
Other _____ |

Evaluate your sleep last night.
Scale : 0 1 2 3 4 5   (poor 0 to excellent 5)
Bad or disturbing dreams?_____

Dizziness? y/n _____
Falls? y/n _____
Depression? y/n _____   Alcohol? y/n
Hallucinations? y/n _____   How much?_____

Did you exercise today? y/n How Long? _____ minutes
Type of Exercise: _____

Did you eat three balanced healthy meals today?
Breakfast y/n _____
Lunch y/n _____
Dinner y/n _____

What did you accomplish today? _____
_____

Date:_____   **Daily Log**   Overall Rating: 😊 😐 ☹

| Did you remember to take your medications today?

_____am/pm y/n
_____am/pm y/n
_____am/pm y/n
_____am/pm y/n
_____am/pm y/n | Off times: Time of day symptoms started: _____

Symptoms: Fatigue, Tremors, Mood Change, Sweating, Anxiety, Not Thinking Clearly, Feeling Restless (circle any that apply)
Other _____ |

Evaluate your sleep last night.
Scale : 0 1 2 3 4 5 (poor 0 to excellent 5)
Bad or disturbing dreams?_____

Dizziness? y/n _____
Falls? y/n _____
Depression? y/n _____   Alcohol? y/n
Hallucinations? y/n _____   How much?_____

Did you exercise today? y/n How Long? _____ minutes
Type of Exercise: _____

Did you eat three balanced healthy meals today?
Breakfast y/n _____
Lunch y/n _____
Dinner y/n _____

What did you accomplish today? _____
_____

Date:_____ **Daily Log** Overall Rating: 😊 😐 ☹

| Did you remember to take your medications today?

_____am/pm y/n
_____am/pm y/n
_____am/pm y/n
_____am/pm y/n
_____am/pm y/n | Off times: Time of day symptoms started: _____

Symptoms: Fatigue, Tremors, Mood Change, Sweating, Anxiety, Not Thinking Clearly, Feeling Restless (circle any that apply)
Other _____ |

Evaluate your sleep last night.
Scale : 0 1 2 3 4 5   (poor 0 to excellent 5)
Bad or disturbing dreams?_____

Dizziness? y/n _____
Falls? y/n _____
Depression? y/n _____   Alcohol? y/n
Hallucinations? y/n _____   How much?_____

Did you exercise today? y/n How Long? _____ minutes
Type of Exercise: _____

Did you eat three balanced healthy meals today?
Breakfast y/n _____
Lunch y/n _____
Dinner y/n _____

What did you accomplish today? _____
_____

Date:_____ **Daily Log** Overall Rating: 😊 😐 ☹️

| Did you remember to take your medications today?

_____am/pm y/n
_____am/pm y/n
_____am/pm y/n
_____am/pm y/n
_____am/pm y/n | Off times: Time of day symptoms started: _____

Symptoms: Fatigue, Tremors, Mood Change, Sweating, Anxiety, Not Thinking Clearly, Feeling Restless (circle any that apply)
Other _____ |

Evaluate your sleep last night.
Scale : 0 1 2 3 4 5   (poor 0 to excellent 5)
Bad or disturbing dreams?_____

Dizziness? y/n _____
Falls? y/n _____
Depression? y/n _____   Alcohol? y/n
Hallucinations? y/n _____   How much?_____

Did you exercise today? y/n How Long? _____ minutes
Type of Exercise: _____

Did you eat three balanced healthy meals today?
Breakfast y/n _____
Lunch y/n _____
Dinner y/n _____

What did you accomplish today? _____
_____

Date:_____ **Daily Log** Overall Rating: 😊 😐 ☹️

| Did you remember to take your medications today?

_____am/pm y/n
_____am/pm y/n
_____am/pm y/n
_____am/pm y/n
_____am/pm y/n | Off times: Time of day symptoms started: _____

Symptoms: Fatigue, Tremors, Mood Change, Sweating, Anxiety, Not Thinking Clearly, Feeling Restless (circle any that apply)
Other _____ |

Evaluate your sleep last night.
Scale : 0 1 2 3 4 5 (poor 0 to excellent 5)
Bad or disturbing dreams?_____

Dizziness? y/n _____
Falls? y/n _____
Depression? y/n _____   Alcohol? y/n
Hallucinations? y/n _____   How much?_____

Did you exercise today? y/n How Long? _____ minutes
Type of Exercise: _____

Did you eat three balanced healthy meals today?
Breakfast y/n _____
Lunch y/n _____
Dinner y/n _____

What did you accomplish today? _____
_____

Date:_____ **Daily Log** Overall Rating: 😊 😐 ☹

| Did you remember to take your medications today?

_____am/pm y/n
_____am/pm y/n
_____am/pm y/n
_____am/pm y/n
_____am/pm y/n | Off times: Time of day symptoms started: _____

Symptoms: Fatigue, Tremors, Mood Change, Sweating, Anxiety, Not Thinking Clearly, Feeling Restless (circle any that apply)
Other _____ |

Evaluate your sleep last night.
Scale : 0 1 2 3 4 5 (poor 0 to excellent 5)
Bad or disturbing dreams?_____

Dizziness? y/n _____
Falls? y/n _____
Depression? y/n _____   Alcohol? y/n
Hallucinations? y/n _____   How much?_____

Did you exercise today? y/n How Long? _____ minutes
Type of Exercise: _____

Did you eat three balanced healthy meals today?
Breakfast y/n _____
Lunch y/n _____
Dinner y/n _____

What did you accomplish today? _____
_____

Date:_____   **Daily Log**   Overall Rating: ☺ 😐 ☹

Did you remember to take your medications today?	Off times: Time of day symptoms started: _____
_____am/pm y/n _____am/pm y/n _____am/pm y/n _____am/pm y/n _____am/pm y/n	Symptoms: Fatigue, Tremors, Mood Change, Sweating, Anxiety, Not Thinking Clearly, Feeling Restless (circle any that apply) Other _____

Evaluate your sleep last night.
Scale : 0 1 2 3 4 5 (poor 0 to excellent 5)
Bad or disturbing dreams?_____

Dizziness? y/n _____
Falls? y/n _____
Depression? y/n _____   Alcohol? y/n
Hallucinations? y/n _____   How much?_____

Did you exercise today? y/n How Long? _____ minutes
Type of Exercise: _____

Did you eat three balanced healthy meals today?
Breakfast y/n _____
Lunch y/n _____
Dinner y/n _____

What did you accomplish today? _____
_____

Date:_____ **Daily Log** Overall Rating: 😊 😐 ☹️

Did you remember to take your medications today?	Off times: Time of day symptoms started: _____
_____am/pm y/n _____am/pm y/n _____am/pm y/n _____am/pm y/n _____am/pm y/n	Symptoms: Fatigue, Tremors, Mood Change, Sweating, Anxiety, Not Thinking Clearly, Feeling Restless (circle any that apply) Other _____

Evaluate your sleep last night.
Scale : 0 1 2 3 4 5 (poor 0 to excellent 5)
Bad or disturbing dreams?_____

Dizziness? y/n _____
Falls? y/n _____
Depression? y/n _____   Alcohol? y/n
Hallucinations? y/n _____   How much?_____

Did you exercise today? y/n How Long? _____ minutes
Type of Exercise: _____

Did you eat three balanced healthy meals today?
Breakfast y/n _____
Lunch y/n _____
Dinner y/n _____

What did you accomplish today? _____
_____

Date:_____ **Daily Log** Overall Rating: 😊 😐 ☹

Did you remember to take your medications today?

_____am/pm y/n
_____am/pm y/n
_____am/pm y/n
_____am/pm y/n
_____am/pm y/n

Off times: Time of day symptoms started: _____

Symptoms: Fatigue, Tremors, Mood Change, Sweating, Anxiety, Not Thinking Clearly, Feeling Restless (circle any that apply)
Other _____

Evaluate your sleep last night.
Scale : 0 1 2 3 4 5 (poor 0 to excellent 5)
Bad or disturbing dreams?_____

Dizziness? y/n _____
Falls? y/n _____
Depression? y/n _____   Alcohol? y/n
Hallucinations? y/n _____   How much?_____

Did you exercise today? y/n How Long? _____ minutes
Type of Exercise: _____

Did you eat three balanced healthy meals today?
Breakfast y/n _____
Lunch y/n _____
Dinner y/n _____

What did you accomplish today? _____
_____

Date:_____   **Daily Log**   Overall Rating: 😊 😐 ☹

| Did you remember to take your medications today?

_____am/pm y/n
_____am/pm y/n
_____am/pm y/n
_____am/pm y/n
_____am/pm y/n | Off times: Time of day symptoms started: _____

Symptoms: Fatigue, Tremors, Mood Change, Sweating, Anxiety, Not Thinking Clearly, Feeling Restless (circle any that apply)
Other _____ |

Evaluate your sleep last night.
Scale : 0 1 2 3 4 5   (poor 0 to excellent 5)
Bad or disturbing dreams?_____

Dizziness? y/n _____
Falls? y/n _____
Depression? y/n _____   Alcohol? y/n
Hallucinations? y/n _____   How much?_____

Did you exercise today? y/n How Long? _____ minutes
Type of Exercise: _____

Did you eat three balanced healthy meals today?
Breakfast y/n _____
Lunch y/n _____
Dinner y/n _____

What did you accomplish today? _____
_____

Date:_____ **Daily Log** Overall Rating: ☺ 😐 ☹

Did you remember to take your medications today?

_____am/pm y/n
_____am/pm y/n
_____am/pm y/n
_____am/pm y/n
_____am/pm y/n

Off times: Time of day symptoms started: _____

Symptoms: Fatigue, Tremors, Mood Change, Sweating, Anxiety, Not Thinking Clearly, Feeling Restless (circle any that apply)
Other _____

Evaluate your sleep last night.
Scale : 0 1 2 3 4 5 (poor 0 to excellent 5)
Bad or disturbing dreams?_____

Dizziness? y/n _____
Falls? y/n _____
Depression? y/n _____   Alcohol? y/n
Hallucinations? y/n _____ How much?_____

Did you exercise today? y/n How Long? _____ minutes
Type of Exercise: _____

Did you eat three balanced healthy meals today?
Breakfast y/n _____
Lunch y/n _____
Dinner y/n _____

What did you accomplish today? _____
_____

Date:_____ **Daily Log** Overall Rating: 🙂 😐 ☹️

| Did you remember to take your medications today?

_____am/pm y/n
_____am/pm y/n
_____am/pm y/n
_____am/pm y/n
_____am/pm y/n | Off times: Time of day symptoms started: _____

Symptoms: Fatigue, Tremors, Mood Change, Sweating, Anxiety, Not Thinking Clearly, Feeling Restless (circle any that apply)
Other _____ |

Evaluate your sleep last night.
Scale : 0 1 2 3 4 5 (poor 0 to excellent 5)
Bad or disturbing dreams?_____

Dizziness? y/n _____
Falls? y/n _____
Depression? y/n _____   Alcohol? y/n
Hallucinations? y/n _____   How much?_____

Did you exercise today? y/n How Long? _____ minutes
Type of Exercise: _____

Did you eat three balanced healthy meals today?
Breakfast y/n _____
Lunch y/n _____
Dinner y/n _____

What did you accomplish today? _____
_____

Date:_____ **Daily Log** Overall Rating: 😊 😐 ☹

| Did you remember to take your medications today?

_____am/pm y/n
_____am/pm y/n
_____am/pm y/n
_____am/pm y/n
_____am/pm y/n | Off times: Time of day symptoms started: _____

Symptoms: Fatigue, Tremors, Mood Change, Sweating, Anxiety, Not Thinking Clearly, Feeling Restless (circle any that apply)
Other _____ |

Evaluate your sleep last night.
Scale : 0 1 2 3 4 5 (poor 0 to excellent 5)
Bad or disturbing dreams?_____

Dizziness? y/n _____
Falls? y/n _____
Depression? y/n _____   Alcohol? y/n
Hallucinations? y/n _____   How much?_____

Did you exercise today? y/n How Long? _____ minutes
Type of Exercise: _____

Did you eat three balanced healthy meals today?
Breakfast y/n _____
Lunch y/n _____
Dinner y/n _____

What did you accomplish today? _____
_____

Date:_____ **Daily Log** Overall Rating: 😊 😐 ☹

Did you remember to take your medications today?	Off times: Time of day symptoms started: _____
_____am/pm y/n _____am/pm y/n _____am/pm y/n _____am/pm y/n _____am/pm y/n	Symptoms: Fatigue, Tremors, Mood Change, Sweating, Anxiety, Not Thinking Clearly, Feeling Restless (circle any that apply) Other _____

Evaluate your sleep last night.
Scale : 0 1 2 3 4 5 (poor 0 to excellent 5)
Bad or disturbing dreams?_____

Dizziness? y/n _____
Falls? y/n _____
Depression? y/n _____   Alcohol? y/n
Hallucinations? y/n _____   How much?_____

Did you exercise today? y/n How Long? _____ minutes
Type of Exercise: _____

Did you eat three balanced healthy meals today?
Breakfast y/n _____
Lunch y/n _____
Dinner y/n _____

What did you accomplish today? _____
_____

Date:_____ **Daily Log**   Overall Rating: 😊 😐 ☹

| Did you remember to take your medications today?

_____am/pm y/n
_____am/pm y/n
_____am/pm y/n
_____am/pm y/n
_____am/pm y/n | Off times: Time of day symptoms started: _____

Symptoms: Fatigue, Tremors, Mood Change, Sweating, Anxiety, Not Thinking Clearly, Feeling Restless (circle any that apply)
Other _____ |

Evaluate your sleep last night.
Scale : 0 1 2 3 4 5   (poor 0 to excellent 5)
Bad or disturbing dreams?_____

Dizziness? y/n _____
Falls? y/n _____
Depression? y/n _____   Alcohol? y/n
Hallucinations? y/n _____   How much?_____

Did you exercise today? y/n How Long? _____ minutes
Type of Exercise: _____

Did you eat three balanced healthy meals today?
Breakfast y/n _____
Lunch y/n _____
Dinner y/n _____

What did you accomplish today? _____
_____

Date:_____   **Daily Log**   Overall Rating: 😊 😐 ☹

| Did you remember to take your medications today?

_____am/pm y/n
_____am/pm y/n
_____am/pm y/n
_____am/pm y/n
_____am/pm y/n | Off times: Time of day symptoms started: _____

Symptoms: Fatigue, Tremors, Mood Change, Sweating, Anxiety, Not Thinking Clearly, Feeling Restless (circle any that apply)
Other _____ |

Evaluate your sleep last night.
Scale : 0 1 2 3 4 5   (poor 0 to excellent 5)
Bad or disturbing dreams?_____

Dizziness? y/n _____
Falls? y/n _____
Depression? y/n _____   Alcohol? y/n
Hallucinations? y/n _____   How much?_____

Did you exercise today? y/n How Long? _____ minutes
Type of Exercise: _____

Did you eat three balanced healthy meals today?
Breakfast y/n _____
Lunch y/n _____
Dinner y/n _____

What did you accomplish today? _____
_____

Date:_____ **Daily Log** Overall Rating: 😊 😐 ☹

| Did you remember to take your medications today?

_____am/pm y/n
_____am/pm y/n
_____am/pm y/n
_____am/pm y/n
_____am/pm y/n | Off times: Time of day symptoms started: _____

Symptoms: Fatigue, Tremors, Mood Change, Sweating, Anxiety, Not Thinking Clearly, Feeling Restless (circle any that apply)
Other _____ |

Evaluate your sleep last night.
Scale : 0 1 2 3 4 5   (poor 0 to excellent 5)
Bad or disturbing dreams?_____

Dizziness? y/n _____
Falls? y/n _____
Depression? y/n _____   Alcohol? y/n
Hallucinations? y/n _____   How much?_____

Did you exercise today? y/n How Long? _____ minutes
Type of Exercise: _____

Did you eat three balanced healthy meals today?
Breakfast y/n _____
Lunch y/n _____
Dinner y/n _____

What did you accomplish today? _____
_____

Date:_____   **Daily Log**   Overall Rating: 🙂 😐 ☹️

Did you remember to take your medications today?

_____am/pm y/n
_____am/pm y/n
_____am/pm y/n
_____am/pm y/n
_____am/pm y/n

Off times: Time of day symptoms started: _____

Symptoms: Fatigue, Tremors, Mood Change, Sweating, Anxiety, Not Thinking Clearly, Feeling Restless (circle any that apply)
Other _____

Evaluate your sleep last night.
Scale : 0 1 2 3 4 5   (poor 0 to excellent 5)
Bad or disturbing dreams?_____

Dizziness? y/n _____
Falls? y/n _____
Depression? y/n _____   Alcohol? y/n
Hallucinations? y/n _____   How much?_____

Did you exercise today? y/n How Long? _____ minutes
Type of Exercise: _____

Did you eat three balanced healthy meals today?
Breakfast y/n _____
Lunch y/n _____
Dinner y/n _____

What did you accomplish today? _____
_____

Date:_____   **Daily Log**   Overall Rating: 😊 😐 ☹

| Did you remember to take your medications today? _____am/pm y/n _____am/pm y/n _____am/pm y/n _____am/pm y/n _____am/pm y/n | Off times: Time of day symptoms started: _____ Symptoms: Fatigue, Tremors, Mood Change, Sweating, Anxiety, Not Thinking Clearly, Feeling Restless (circle any that apply) Other _____ |

Evaluate your sleep last night.
Scale : 0 1 2 3 4 5 (poor 0 to excellent 5)
Bad or disturbing dreams?_____

Dizziness? y/n _____
Falls? y/n _____
Depression? y/n _____   Alcohol? y/n
Hallucinations? y/n _____   How much?_____

Did you exercise today? y/n How Long? _____ minutes
Type of Exercise: _____

Did you eat three balanced healthy meals today?
Breakfast y/n _____
Lunch y/n _____
Dinner y/n _____

What did you accomplish today? _____
_____

Date:_____   **Daily Log**   Overall Rating: 😊 😐 ☹️

| Did you remember to take your medications today?

_____am/pm y/n
_____am/pm y/n
_____am/pm y/n
_____am/pm y/n
_____am/pm y/n | Off times: Time of day symptoms started: _____

Symptoms: Fatigue, Tremors, Mood Change, Sweating, Anxiety, Not Thinking Clearly, Feeling Restless (circle any that apply)
Other _____ |

Evaluate your sleep last night.
Scale : 0 1 2 3 4 5 (poor 0 to excellent 5)
Bad or disturbing dreams?_____

Dizziness? y/n _____
Falls? y/n _____
Depression? y/n _____   Alcohol? y/n
Hallucinations? y/n _____   How much?_____

Did you exercise today? y/n How Long? _____ minutes
Type of Exercise: _____

Did you eat three balanced healthy meals today?
Breakfast y/n _____
Lunch y/n _____
Dinner y/n _____

What did you accomplish today? _____
_____

Date:_____   **Daily Log**   Overall Rating: 😊 😐 ☹️

| Did you remember to take your medications today? _____am/pm y/n _____am/pm y/n _____am/pm y/n _____am/pm y/n _____am/pm y/n | Off times: Time of day symptoms started: _____ Symptoms: Fatigue, Tremors, Mood Change, Sweating, Anxiety, Not Thinking Clearly, Feeling Restless (circle any that apply) Other _____ |

Evaluate your sleep last night.
Scale : 0 1 2 3 4 5 (poor 0 to excellent 5)
Bad or disturbing dreams?_____

Dizziness? y/n _____
Falls? y/n _____
Depression? y/n _____   Alcohol? y/n
Hallucinations? y/n _____   How much?_____

Did you exercise today? y/n How Long? _____ minutes
Type of Exercise: _____

Did you eat three balanced healthy meals today?
Breakfast y/n _____
Lunch y/n _____
Dinner y/n _____

What did you accomplish today? _____
_____

Date:_____   **Daily Log**   Overall Rating: 😊 😐 ☹

Did you remember to take your medications today?	Off times: Time of day symptoms started: _____
_____am/pm y/n _____am/pm y/n _____am/pm y/n _____am/pm y/n _____am/pm y/n	Symptoms: Fatigue, Tremors, Mood Change, Sweating, Anxiety, Not Thinking Clearly, Feeling Restless (circle any that apply) Other _____

Evaluate your sleep last night.
Scale : 0 1 2 3 4 5 (poor 0 to excellent 5)
Bad or disturbing dreams?_____

Dizziness? y/n _____
Falls? y/n _____
Depression? y/n _____   Alcohol? y/n
Hallucinations? y/n _____   How much?_____

Did you exercise today? y/n How Long? _____ minutes
Type of Exercise: _____

Did you eat three balanced healthy meals today?
Breakfast y/n _____
Lunch y/n _____
Dinner y/n _____

What did you accomplish today? _____
_____

Date:_____   **Daily Log**   Overall Rating: 😊 😐 ☹

| Did you remember to take your medications today?

_____am/pm y/n
_____am/pm y/n
_____am/pm y/n
_____am/pm y/n
_____am/pm y/n | Off times: Time of day symptoms started: _____

Symptoms: Fatigue, Tremors, Mood Change, Sweating, Anxiety, Not Thinking Clearly, Feeling Restless (circle any that apply)
Other _____ |

Evaluate your sleep last night.
Scale : 0 1 2 3 4 5   (poor 0 to excellent 5)
Bad or disturbing dreams?_____

Dizziness? y/n _____
Falls? y/n _____
Depression? y/n _____   Alcohol? y/n
Hallucinations? y/n _____   How much?_____

Did you exercise today? y/n How Long? _____ minutes
Type of Exercise: _____

Did you eat three balanced healthy meals today?
Breakfast y/n _____
Lunch y/n _____
Dinner y/n _____

What did you accomplish today? _____
_____

Date:_____ **Daily Log** Overall Rating: 😊 😐 ☹️

| Did you remember to take your medications today? _____am/pm y/n _____am/pm y/n _____am/pm y/n _____am/pm y/n _____am/pm y/n | Off times: Time of day symptoms started: _____ Symptoms: Fatigue, Tremors, Mood Change, Sweating, Anxiety, Not Thinking Clearly, Feeling Restless (circle any that apply) Other _____ |

Evaluate your sleep last night.
Scale : 0 1 2 3 4 5 (poor 0 to excellent 5)
Bad or disturbing dreams?_____

Dizziness? y/n _____
Falls? y/n _____
Depression? y/n _____   Alcohol? y/n
Hallucinations? y/n _____   How much?_____

Did you exercise today? y/n How Long? _____ minutes
Type of Exercise: _____

Did you eat three balanced healthy meals today?
Breakfast y/n _____
Lunch y/n _____
Dinner y/n _____

What did you accomplish today? _____
_____

Date:_____ **Daily Log**   Overall Rating: ☺ 😐 ☹

| Did you remember to take your medications today? _____am/pm y/n _____am/pm y/n _____am/pm y/n _____am/pm y/n _____am/pm y/n | Off times: Time of day symptoms started: _____ Symptoms: Fatigue, Tremors, Mood Change, Sweating, Anxiety, Not Thinking Clearly, Feeling Restless (circle any that apply) Other _____ |

Evaluate your sleep last night.
Scale : 0 1 2 3 4 5   (poor 0 to excellent 5)
Bad or disturbing dreams?_____

Dizziness? y/n _____
Falls? y/n _____
Depression? y/n _____   Alcohol? y/n
Hallucinations? y/n _____   How much?_____

Did you exercise today? y/n How Long? _____ minutes
Type of Exercise: _____

Did you eat three balanced healthy meals today?
Breakfast y/n _____
Lunch y/n _____
Dinner y/n _____

What did you accomplish today? _____
_____

Date:_____   **Daily Log**   Overall Rating: 😊 😐 ☹

Did you remember to take your medications today?	Off times: Time of day symptoms started: _____
_____am/pm y/n _____am/pm y/n _____am/pm y/n _____am/pm y/n _____am/pm y/n	Symptoms: Fatigue, Tremors, Mood Change, Sweating, Anxiety, Not Thinking Clearly, Feeling Restless (circle any that apply) Other _____

Evaluate your sleep last night.
Scale : 0 1 2 3 4 5 (poor 0 to excellent 5)
Bad or disturbing dreams?_____

Dizziness? y/n _____
Falls? y/n _____
Depression? y/n _____   Alcohol? y/n
Hallucinations? y/n _____   How much?_____

Did you exercise today? y/n How Long? _____ minutes
Type of Exercise: _____

Did you eat three balanced healthy meals today?
Breakfast y/n _____
Lunch y/n _____
Dinner y/n _____

What did you accomplish today? _____
_____

Date:_____ **Daily Log** Overall Rating: ☺ 😐 ☹

| Did you remember to take your medications today?

_____am/pm y/n
_____am/pm y/n
_____am/pm y/n
_____am/pm y/n
_____am/pm y/n | Off times: Time of day symptoms started: _____

Symptoms: Fatigue, Tremors, Mood Change, Sweating, Anxiety, Not Thinking Clearly, Feeling Restless (circle any that apply)
Other _____ |

Evaluate your sleep last night.
Scale : 0 1 2 3 4 5   (poor 0 to excellent 5)
Bad or disturbing dreams?_____

Dizziness? y/n _____
Falls? y/n _____
Depression? y/n _____   Alcohol? y/n
Hallucinations? y/n _____   How much?_____

Did you exercise today? y/n How Long? _____ minutes
Type of Exercise: _____

Did you eat three balanced healthy meals today?
Breakfast y/n _____
Lunch y/n _____
Dinner y/n _____

What did you accomplish today? _____
_____

Date:_____ **Daily Log** Overall Rating: 😊 😐 ☹️

| Did you remember to take your medications today?

_____am/pm y/n
_____am/pm y/n
_____am/pm y/n
_____am/pm y/n
_____am/pm y/n | Off times: Time of day symptoms started: _____

Symptoms: Fatigue, Tremors, Mood Change, Sweating, Anxiety, Not Thinking Clearly, Feeling Restless (circle any that apply)
Other _____ |

Evaluate your sleep last night.
Scale : 0 1 2 3 4 5   (poor 0 to excellent 5)
Bad or disturbing dreams?_____

Dizziness? y/n _____
Falls? y/n _____
Depression? y/n _____   Alcohol? y/n
Hallucinations? y/n _____   How much?_____

Did you exercise today? y/n How Long? _____ minutes
Type of Exercise: _____

Did you eat three balanced healthy meals today?
Breakfast y/n _____
Lunch y/n _____
Dinner y/n _____

What did you accomplish today? _____
_____

Date:_____   **Daily Log**   Overall Rating: 😊 😐 ☹

| Did you remember to take your medications today?

_____am/pm y/n
_____am/pm y/n
_____am/pm y/n
_____am/pm y/n
_____am/pm y/n | Off times: Time of day symptoms started: _____

Symptoms: Fatigue, Tremors, Mood Change, Sweating, Anxiety, Not Thinking Clearly, Feeling Restless (circle any that apply)
Other _____ |

Evaluate your sleep last night.
Scale : 0 1 2 3 4 5   (poor 0 to excellent 5)
Bad or disturbing dreams?_____

Dizziness? y/n _____
Falls? y/n _____
Depression? y/n _____   Alcohol? y/n
Hallucinations? y/n _____   How much?_____

Did you exercise today? y/n How Long? _____ minutes
Type of Exercise: _____

Did you eat three balanced healthy meals today?
Breakfast y/n _____
Lunch y/n _____
Dinner y/n _____

What did you accomplish today? _____
_____

Date:_____   **Daily Log**   Overall Rating: 🙂 😐 ☹

Did you remember to take your medications today?	Off times: Time of day symptoms started: _____
_____am/pm y/n _____am/pm y/n _____am/pm y/n _____am/pm y/n _____am/pm y/n	Symptoms: Fatigue, Tremors, Mood Change, Sweating, Anxiety, Not Thinking Clearly, Feeling Restless (circle any that apply) Other _____

Evaluate your sleep last night.
Scale : 0 1 2 3 4 5 (poor 0 to excellent 5)
Bad or disturbing dreams?_____

Dizziness? y/n _____
Falls? y/n _____
Depression? y/n _____   Alcohol? y/n
Hallucinations? y/n _____   How much?_____

Did you exercise today? y/n How Long? _____ minutes
Type of Exercise: _____

Did you eat three balanced healthy meals today?
Breakfast y/n _____
Lunch y/n _____
Dinner y/n _____

What did you accomplish today? _____
_____

Date:_____ **Daily Log** Overall Rating: ☺ 😐 ☹

| Did you remember to take your medications today?

_____am/pm y/n
_____am/pm y/n
_____am/pm y/n
_____am/pm y/n
_____am/pm y/n | Off times: Time of day symptoms started: _____

Symptoms: Fatigue, Tremors, Mood Change, Sweating, Anxiety, Not Thinking Clearly, Feeling Restless (circle any that apply)
Other _____ |

Evaluate your sleep last night.
Scale : 0 1 2 3 4 5 (poor 0 to excellent 5)
Bad or disturbing dreams?_____

Dizziness? y/n _____
Falls? y/n _____
Depression? y/n _____   Alcohol? y/n
Hallucinations? y/n _____   How much?_____

Did you exercise today? y/n How Long? _____ minutes
Type of Exercise: _____

Did you eat three balanced healthy meals today?
Breakfast y/n _____
Lunch y/n _____
Dinner y/n _____

What did you accomplish today? _____
_____

Date:_____ **Daily Log** Overall Rating: 😊 😐 ☹

Did you remember to take your medications today? _____am/pm y/n _____am/pm y/n _____am/pm y/n _____am/pm y/n _____am/pm y/n	Off times: Time of day symptoms started: _____ Symptoms: Fatigue, Tremors, Mood Change, Sweating, Anxiety, Not Thinking Clearly, Feeling Restless (circle any that apply) Other _____

Evaluate your sleep last night.
Scale : 0 1 2 3 4 5   (poor 0 to excellent 5)
Bad or disturbing dreams?_____

Dizziness? y/n _____
Falls? y/n _____
Depression? y/n _____   Alcohol? y/n
Hallucinations? y/n _____   How much?_____

Did you exercise today? y/n How Long? _____ minutes
Type of Exercise: _____

Did you eat three balanced healthy meals today?
Breakfast y/n _____
Lunch y/n _____
Dinner y/n _____

What did you accomplish today? _____
_____

Date:_____ **Daily Log** Overall Rating: 😊 😐 ☹️

Did you remember to take your medications today?

_____am/pm y/n
_____am/pm y/n
_____am/pm y/n
_____am/pm y/n
_____am/pm y/n

Off times: Time of day symptoms started: _____

Symptoms: Fatigue, Tremors, Mood Change, Sweating, Anxiety, Not Thinking Clearly, Feeling Restless (circle any that apply)
Other _____

Evaluate your sleep last night.
Scale : 0 1 2 3 4 5 (poor 0 to excellent 5)
Bad or disturbing dreams?_____

Dizziness? y/n _____
Falls? y/n _____
Depression? y/n _____   Alcohol? y/n
Hallucinations? y/n _____   How much?_____

Did you exercise today? y/n How Long? _____ minutes
Type of Exercise: _____

Did you eat three balanced healthy meals today?
Breakfast y/n _____
Lunch y/n _____
Dinner y/n _____

What did you accomplish today? _____
_____

Date:_____ **Daily Log**   Overall Rating: 🙂 😐 ☹

Did you remember to take your medications today?

_____am/pm y/n
_____am/pm y/n
_____am/pm y/n
_____am/pm y/n
_____am/pm y/n

Off times: Time of day symptoms started: _____

Symptoms: Fatigue, Tremors, Mood Change, Sweating, Anxiety, Not Thinking Clearly, Feeling Restless (circle any that apply)
Other _____

Evaluate your sleep last night.
Scale : 0 1 2 3 4 5 (poor 0 to excellent 5)
Bad or disturbing dreams?_____

Dizziness? y/n _____
Falls? y/n _____
Depression? y/n _____   Alcohol? y/n
Hallucinations? y/n _____   How much?_____

Did you exercise today? y/n How Long? _____ minutes
Type of Exercise: _____

Did you eat three balanced healthy meals today?
Breakfast y/n _____
Lunch y/n _____
Dinner y/n _____

What did you accomplish today? _____
_____

Date:_____ **Daily Log** Overall Rating: 😊 😐 ☹️

Did you remember to take your medications today?	Off times: Time of day symptoms started: _____
_____am/pm y/n _____am/pm y/n _____am/pm y/n _____am/pm y/n _____am/pm y/n	Symptoms: Fatigue, Tremors, Mood Change, Sweating, Anxiety, Not Thinking Clearly, Feeling Restless (circle any that apply) Other _____

Evaluate your sleep last night.
Scale : 0 1 2 3 4 5 (poor 0 to excellent 5)
Bad or disturbing dreams?_____

Dizziness? y/n _____
Falls? y/n _____
Depression? y/n _____   Alcohol? y/n
Hallucinations? y/n _____   How much?_____

Did you exercise today? y/n How Long? _____ minutes
Type of Exercise: _____

Did you eat three balanced healthy meals today?
Breakfast y/n _____
Lunch y/n _____
Dinner y/n _____

What did you accomplish today? _____
_____

Date:_____ **Daily Log** Overall Rating: 🙂 😐 ☹

Did you remember to take your medications today?	Off times: Time of day symptoms started: _____
_____am/pm y/n _____am/pm y/n _____am/pm y/n _____am/pm y/n _____am/pm y/n	Symptoms: Fatigue, Tremors, Mood Change, Sweating, Anxiety, Not Thinking Clearly, Feeling Restless (circle any that apply) Other _____

Evaluate your sleep last night.
Scale : 0 1 2 3 4 5 (poor 0 to excellent 5)
Bad or disturbing dreams?_____

Dizziness? y/n _____
Falls? y/n _____
Depression? y/n _____   Alcohol? y/n
Hallucinations? y/n _____   How much?_____

Did you exercise today? y/n How Long? _____ minutes
Type of Exercise: _____

Did you eat three balanced healthy meals today?
Breakfast y/n _____
Lunch y/n _____
Dinner y/n _____

What did you accomplish today? _____
_____

Printed in Great Britain
by Amazon